STRESSES OF MODERN MAN

Mental Health Challenges Explained

Ann Bowditch

Dear Dave,
   You've been a huge help
   Much appreciated
   Ann Bowditch

Orders: To place orders of this book, please visit www.hypnotherapy.gg or e-mail: ann@hypnotherapy.gg

ISBN: 978-1-9160758-2-5

Copyright © 2021 by Ann Bowditch. All rights reserved.

All rights reserved. Apart from any permitted use under UK copyright law, no part of this publication may be reproduced or transmitted in any form or by any means, electronic or mechanical, including photocopying, recording, or any information, storage or retrieval system, without permission in writing from the publisher, Ann Bowditch, or under license from The Copyright Licensing Agency Limited. Further details of such licenses (for reprographic reproduction) may be obtained from The Copyright Licensing Agency Ltd www.cla.co.uk

First Published: 2021

Cover design by Ken Dawson at Creative Covers

Disclaimer

The ideas and opinions in Stresses of Modern Man represent those of Ann Bowditch, the author, as of the date of publication. The author is a holistic health practitioner, specifically qualified in the science and practice of META-Health which focusses on the impact of stress on the body, mind and social health.

The author is also a Clinical Hypnotherapist under the General Hypnotherapy Register and General Hypnotherapy Standards Council. Trained in other therapies, her views and opinions are also based on experience gained through helping clients improve their well-being.

This book is for informational and educational purposes only, to aid and support emotional well-being and personal development. The information in this book should not be treated as a substitute for the medical advice of physicians. You are advised to take full responsibility for yourself at all times and to seek the support of a qualified emotional health practitioner, doctor, health practitioner or therapist if you have any concerns about your physical health or emotional well-being.

If you are suffering from any physical or psychiatric condition, please seek the advice of the appropriately qualified health professional. Any use of information in this book is at the reader's discretion and risk. The author and publisher cannot be held responsible for any loss, claim, or damage arising from the use, or misuse, of the suggestions made, or the failure to take medical advice.

The information herein may be subject to varying laws, regulations and practices in different areas, states and countries. The purchaser and the reader assume full responsibility for the use of the information.

Any perceived slight of specific people or organisations is unintentional.

Any links to other websites or contact details are for information only and are not warranted for content, performance, accuracy or any other implied or explicit purpose.

This book does not reference all mental health issues but provides information to help you understand why mental health issues may have occurred.

The author and publisher do not assume, and hereby disclaim, any liability to any party for any loss, damage or disruption caused by errors or omissions, whether such errors or omissions result from negligence, accident or any other cause by using any of the disclaimers within this book.

If you are suffering mental health issues, please seek professional help.

Contents

INTRODUCTION

1. Let's get started	9
2. About Ann	14
3. Evolution of man	17
4. The truth about mental health	20
5. Back to you	31
6. Steps to change	33
7. Opening up to someone close	38

SECTION 1:
UNDERSTANDING YOURSELF AND WHERE THINGS START TO GO WRONG

8. What you believe is important	43
9. When to seek help	54
10. Should, could, would	56
11. Lack of fulfilment	62
12. The male introvert	65
13. Socialising	70
14. Confidence	73
15. Finances	87
16. Self-acceptance	93
17. Medication	98
18. Childhood abuse	100
19. Relationship issues	109
20. ADHD and ASD	120

SECTION 2:
HOW WE RESPOND TO UNRESOLVED ISSUES

21. Addiction	131
22. Anxiety and panic attacks	143
23. Grief	161
24. Insomnia	178
25. Erectile dysfunction	186
26. Anger and aggression	192
27. Depression	206
28. Post-traumatic stress disorder	218
29. Obsessive-compulsive disorder	220
30. Eating disorders	223
31. Self-harm	229
32. Suicidal thoughts	232

SECTION 3: CREATING GOOD MENTAL HEALTH

33. The road to recovery	241
34. General well-being	243
35. Well-being activities	253
36. Power of the breath	257
37. Affirm the positive	262
38. Seek out the positive	265
39. Social media boundaries	267
40. Use your inner voice wisely	270
41. Visualise what you do want	276
42. Create the life you desire	282
43. Appreciate you	287
44. Positive tapping	291
45. Three words tapping	298
46. Mental health plan	301
47. Therapy options	305
48. My final message	314

APPENDIX

I Communication Form	317
II. Tapping scripts	321
III. Example Health Plan	329
IV. Self-recognition form	332
V. Example letter to younger self	335
VI. Help for suicidal thoughts	336
VII. Contact details for suicidal support	338
VIII. Frequently asked questions	340
Contact and links	342
Dedication	344
Acknowledgements	344

Introduction

1. Let's get started

Whatever situation you are in right now is not where you will be forever. Change is possible. Throughout this book, I will share information with you to help you understand yourself better, guide you to make beneficial changes and provide an insight for anyone who wants to understand more about this subject.

I am a straight talker. I have been told that I pull no punches. Mental health is a massive subject and my aim is to make it as clear and understandable as possible. When you begin to understand your own mental health, the way you think and the feelings you have should make more sense.

Men often carry their worries and burdens quietly. You will have a preconceived idea of what a man is and what he should do. A man should hold back his emotions and provide for his family, as well as protecting them. He should be the emotionally and physically strong one. You experience conflict when you do not fulfil those criteria. This can often lead to problems in terms of mental, emotional or physical health. Now we are in a new world, where you do not need to play that archetypal role of man any longer.

One of my readers commented *"if this book can get even one man to face up to the problems they have ignored, pretended don't exist or which they have 'bloked' away then it will have done a lot."*

Through my work as a therapist, I have helped men suffering from many types of mental health issues. The most common of these being anxiety and depression. Sometimes anxiety is specific, such as social or performance related. Other times it is more general.

Issues such as anxiety and depression link to many other areas including insomnia, weight issues, self-confidence, obsessive-compulsive disorder (OCD), addiction, fears, eating disorders, irritable bowel syndrome (IBS) and other physical health issues, self-harming and self-esteem.

Some men struggle to identify the difficulties they are experiencing. They just know they are not in a good place. We do not always need to get trapped in titles and labels to make life better. There are problems, however, there are also reasons and solutions for them.

Sometimes there are minor differences between men and women's mental health issues. However, the one sizeable difference is that women are usually more open to talking about their problems and how they are feeling. This communication provides them with some release and often results in support or advice being offered.

I have worked with boys as young as six and men into their nineties. This has given me great insight into male mental health; the causes, the symptoms and how to help.

Mental health can strike anyone during their lifetime. No one is immune to the possibility of suffering. Successful people may suffer, and often do, as well as those who appear to have their lives in order. There is no age limit or restriction on class or wealth of people who endure mental health challenges.

Something men often fear is judgement about mental health

issues. You might expect others to think badly of you. You could also believe that if you go to a therapist, they will send you off with a flea in your ear for wasting their time. I want to make abundantly clear; this is absolutely not the case. We acknowledge that mental health issues happen and are very real no matter what gender you are. This is an accepted fact by society. As therapists, our job is to help but never to judge you. A therapist who judges would be in the wrong job.

This is not to say that every single person will be completely understanding of mental health problems. Those who do not understand are most likely ignorant or naive. I know, for example, my 85-year-old mum tells me she does not understand anxiety and yet I point out to her that she does experience anxiety from time to time when she over-worries. In fact, she worries more than most people I know.

Anxiety, depression and other mental health issues have been around for a very long time, they are not a new thing of the 21st century. Mental health issues have different labels now compared to decades ago, when perhaps the labels were less kind and understanding with limited descriptions and terminology.

Clients have come to me with a diagnosis such as personality disorders or bipolar. This sometimes causes them to feel they are inadequate, useless or a lost cause.

I recall one client suffering with bipolar who had a very negative view of themselves because of this diagnosis. They called themselves 'weird' and 'a freak'. I explained to them how a part of the brain called the cortex worked when trauma happened and how this resulted in the manic and depressive response. I also explained how the bipolar was most likely a result of the continuous abuse they had suffered in their childhood. Over time they understood that they were not at fault. Bipolar could potentially happen to anyone else placed in a similar situation.

Your health issues, physical or mental should never define you. This is very important. Most mental health issues occur because of circumstances. However, this does not mean that sufferers are any less capable or intelligent than others. They are exceptional human beings.

There are great therapies that can help you overcome those challenges without needing to go into deep analysis on your thoughts and feelings. When I work with men, they will often find benefit in the discussions we have on life issues aside from the therapy. I help them see things from fresh perspectives that guide them to more helpful views on themselves and life.

I have always enjoyed working with boys or men, whatever the age. I have witnessed great commitment to the process for change from men. There is light at the end of the tunnel.

Because this book is about men, then, naturally, I am talking about men. However, please understand that many of the issues I talk about also relate to women. You are not alone.

How to use this book

Mental health is a huge issue. This fact has made it impossible for me to go into each mental health issue or aspect in great detail. However, this book has been written in order to help you understand yourself better. I would like to think it offers you hope and belief that things can change.

I know they can, I just want you to know it too. It provides a starting point to improving your well-being and therefore your life. Having a note book or some way to capture thoughts, key points and realisations would be useful for you.

You may decide to read this book cover to cover. Alternatively, you could sift through to the pages that relate to the challenges you face. In many ways I see this as a dip in and out book especially once you have read through the first two sections. Section 3: 'creating good mental health' is very important if you are going to help yourself to feel better. Do take the time to work through the exercises or suggested changes. These are going to help you on the path to a better life.

I will post supporting videos for the tapping scripts on my YouTube Channel. Supporting forms will be published on www.abauthor.com.

2. About Ann

Here is a little about me as a person and as a therapist.

I am a competitive and outwardly confident person. I consider myself to be a little like those sweets with a tough exterior and a soft centre.

My competitiveness has mostly been directed into the sport of cycling where I have competed at Commonwealth Games level and am three times National Hill Climb Champion. I was named 'Pocket Rocket' by the Isle of Man press and the nickname stuck.

I am really quite modest about my achievements but realise that when writing a book, you cannot beat around the bush.

In some ways I take that desire to do well, into most things that I do and this includes my work. I became self-employed back in 2009 and work then took priority over cycling.

We all have experiences which help us to understand life in new ways. I believe my background and life experiences have done that well for me.

Very briefly, my sister was born with a cleft lip and palate and was terribly bullied. For various reasons, our entire family was impacted by my sister's challenges. I also experienced bullying from her peers at school. I believe this is the reason I built that tough exterior. I expect my sister's challenges are why I like to stick up for the vulnerable.

Witnessing my sister's differences and subsequent challenges and problems that came with the cleft lip and palate, may be why I also see past our differences and appreciate how incredible people can be despite the challenges they are faced with.

I spent the first part of my working life in finance and was working for Barings when Nick Leeson's fraudulent trading bankrupted the bank in 1995. Some of you have probably never heard of this but it was massive news at the time and a very strange period in my life.

Before I came to be a therapist, I was self-employed as a personal trainer and it was that which strangely led me to become a therapist, as people would say "if only you could hypnotise me not to eat the chocolate" or similar comments. I do believe that being a therapist was meant to be. The role seems to fit me like a glove.

I consider myself a 'modern day therapist'. Certain things are important in how I like to work. These include, treating every single person as an individual (I loathe the 'one-size fits all' therapeutic approaches) and really understanding my clients and their challenges. When people work with me it is a joint effort. This is empowering as you find most of the solutions and I just guide you. Teamwork is the way to go.

Importantly I want my clients and readers to feel empowered, obtain a high level of self-worth and gain insight into why they have struggled. I believe knowledge is power.

Sometimes people tell me they think they are weird. I embrace 'weird'. I expect many people think I am weird. I don't care. Embrace the weirdness. What and who is 'normal' anyway?

I am passionate about my work. I really want to help people. Therapy does not always have to be all serious. Very often, with my clients, we can have a giggle and in fact some of my clients find this a big help. My studio has a very warm and inviting atmosphere. One of my clients calls it 'my little sanctuary' and I do feel that describes it perfectly.

I believe strongly that it is imperative to work with the subconscious mind to recover fully because this is where memories, beliefs, habits and behaviours are stored. Coupled with the energy techniques I use; this is powerful work.

I am an empath which means I tend to be able to put myself in your position and imagine what it would be like to have the experiences you have. I do believe this really helps me to work out what needs to change for my clients to recover.

When I work with clients, my aim is for them to finish their course of sessions when they feel in a really good place filled with confidence, self-esteem, self-worth and ready to conquer life.

I wrote my first book because I realised that I was repeating some messages to clients and a book could get those messages out to a wider audience. This was with a view to helping more people. I really enjoyed the process of writing and now, you are reading my third book, written during the Covid-19 pandemic, which caused a worldwide lockdown in 2020.

Writing has become a passion. It enables me to share my knowledge and I would like to think I offer up something new in the world of self-help.

3. Evolution of man

How man and life have evolved is a fundamental factor in why men's mental health has come to the fore.

Let us take a step back a few thousand years. Going back to our ancestry, a man's job was to hunt for food and provide protection for his community. These tasks were straightforward, required little or no instruction and no emotion. The fight or flight response (which I will talk about later) was very useful when you had to either fight off a wild animal or run as fast as you could to save your own life.

Although not luxurious, life was simple way back then. You knew what your job entailed, your physical structure supported this and emotions were unnecessary because of the simplicity of life.

Fast forward to modern times, things have changed in so many ways. Society requires us to engage so much more with others. We have families, friends and colleagues. Social life is busy with little 'down time'. Work is demanding. Often there is too much to do and too few hours to do it in. You feel pressured to perform in many areas of life.

Many families are split. There are separations and divorces, ex's, blended families and stepchildren. It can be difficult keeping the peace and everyone happy.

There are financial strains with high mortgages or rents. You may pay maintenance for your children. The Government reminds you to save for your future when you struggle to make ends meet now. Your children are stressed with friendships, schoolwork or exams. They also have emotional struggles and may experience anxiety, depression, OCD or other issues.

The news and social media are constantly reminding you of just how messed up the world is. You think that everyone else is doing better than you. Your partner is anxious, depressed or suffering in other ways. Elderly parents need caring for. We are confronted with other people's problems.

Because men are the hunter-gatherers, they believe they are the ones who should be able to keep everyone safe and put everything right. Given the above reality check, all I can say is good luck with that.

Whilst all of this is going on, your fight or flight response is being triggered frequently. It exhausts you and yet you cannot sleep because your body is overloaded with stress hormones. This results in you becoming even more exhausted.

I realise that not all the above will relate to you but some will hit home. When stress builds it has to go somewhere. This impacts health in three possible ways: mental, emotional or physical. Our bodies are still functioning as if back in the hunter-gatherer era. You could say we have not evolved physically, mentally or emotionally at the same speed that life has, yet somehow, we are required to function.

I was born in the 1970s and looking back, I can see that life was simpler. My dad was a manager in the book printing section of our local press. I do not recall him discussing work, and he did not appear stressed about it. I do not get the impression he thought about work after he left there at 4 pm Monday to Friday. Mum had cooked dinner, which he had within minutes of walking in through the door. He then spent the evening watching television or sometimes doing DIY. Initially, we could watch one of any three channels and then in 1982 Channel 4 was launched. There was not even a remote control to lose. Our lifestyle was a fair representation of many families.

There were few after-school clubs. I attended Monday Club. I did Brownies for one evening and hated it so never went back. Homework was bearable and not too intrusive.

We were a one-car family. We never went away on holiday as a family. We knew our parents did not have money to throw at us, but we never felt we were living on the breadline either. The best thing is we had no social media or mobile phones. I am so grateful that I grew up in that era, before technology reached the level it has now.

Life happened at a slower pace and seemed so much simpler than it does now. It was not easy, but was different and less complicated. We were more carefree than most people are today.

My message to you is not to give yourself a hard time because there is a lot to deal with in life. It is important to decide what aspects of life you can deal with and change and what areas are not your responsibility.

4. The truth about mental health

It is important to gain a better understanding of mental health issues and why they occur. This is a key factor in beginning the process of being kinder to yourself, which leads to self-acceptance.

When we go through times of stress in our lives, many of us bottle up that stress. We internalise what has happened and run it over and over in our minds. Then we torment ourselves with it all. Add to this the fact that our subconscious mind has stored all the information related to the stress.

People often think the subconscious mind is strange or mystical but it is quite straightforward. First, let's look at the difference between conscious and subconscious.

Conscious means to be aware of or to have knowledge of. For example, if I told you to touch your ear, you would do that action consciously. You would be aware of touching your ear.

Subconscious means below consciousness or without conscious awareness. Another term for this is unconscious. This means to take action that you are not aware of. Most of your daily actions are unconscious. We breathe unconsciously, our heart beats unconsciously and we digest food unconsciously. When you do focused breathing, then it becomes conscious.

Perhaps you remember learning to drive a car. At first all your actions were conscious. You had to concentrate and think about braking, pushing the clutch in and out and accelerating. However, as you became more accustomed to this you would do these actions unconsciously. The same goes for most, if not all, new skills we learn such as a sport or learning to play an instrument. Things become easier when they become unconscious.

Your subconscious mind is the equivalent of a vast database containing information about you and your life. It has stored inside it, every event that has ever happened to you, every conversation you have had, your likes and dislikes, behaviour learned from others, beliefs, values, habits and much more. Imagine a memory stick full of information about you and your life. This is what the subconscious is like.

We process information via the subconscious mind. By accessing the subconscious through hypnotherapy or other techniques, we can bring greater understanding to problems, find solutions and create a positive future. In fact, 95% of mental processing is subconscious and only 5% conscious.

If the stress or trauma we experience is short-lived and not massively severe, such as an argument with the person handling your bank account over a mistake that they have made which gets resolved, then life can usually return to normality, by the following day at the latest, once you have calmed down. However, if this stress is prolonged or severe, there is huge internal processing taking place. Internal processing is both the conscious and subconscious mind making sense of what happened.

You may also be running over worst-case scenarios of how this situation may progress whilst trying to search for a solution. These parts of the mind are trying to achieve clarity and pave the way to move forward so everything can be okay again. The subconscious mind does this in the background. Dreaming is part of the subconscious's way of making sense of events, as weird as some of our dreams can be.

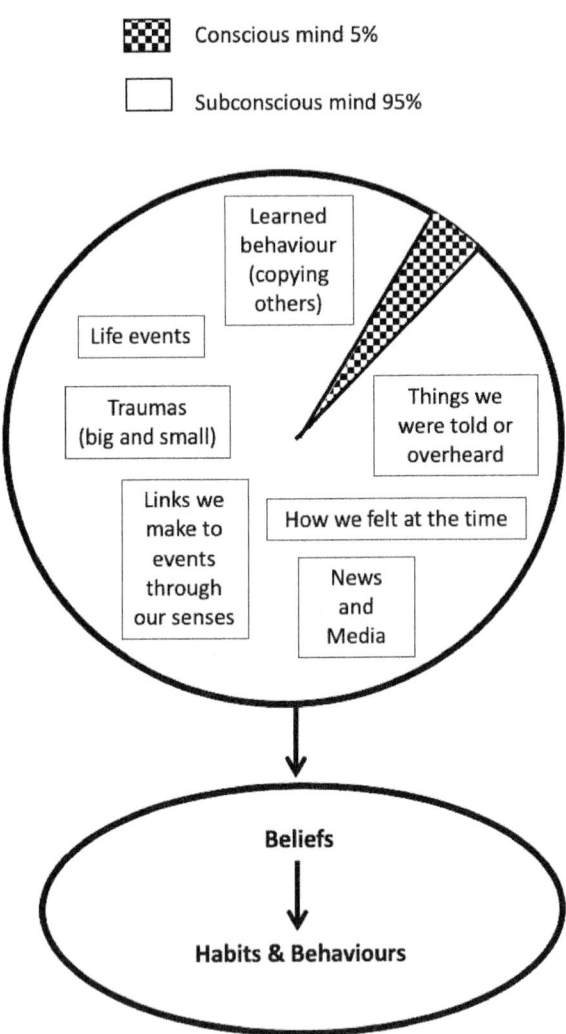

Figure 1: The subconscious mind contains a vast amount of information and acts upon that information creating beliefs that then impact how you see yourself, the world at large and others.

This stress is also held in the cells of our bodies which is why, after stress we are often ill. The obvious example of this is in the run-up to Christmas when so many people are stressed. At work you are trying to keep clients happy and complete all your work before the Christmas break. Colleagues are stressed and this may be impacting on your own stress levels. You may need to work late some nights. At home, people are frantically trying to make the perfect Christmas. Tempers are short. Everyone is tired because of socialising, late nights and eating less healthily than usual.

When you take your Christmas holiday, you come down with some sort of cold or, dare I say, man flu. This is because you have finally allowed your body to take a break and start to recover from the pre-Christmas onslaught. In recovery is when most symptoms flare up. Your body has finally had the go ahead to release all the built-up stress and it usually comes out in some sort of cold or flu.

Stress has to come out in some way. Sometimes stress shows up in a physical form such as flu, irritable bowel syndrome, fatigue, tonsillitis or other physical issues. Other times it shows up through mental health issues such as anxiety and depression or any other plethora of issues including obsessive-compulsive disorder, addiction or self-harm.

Whatever mental health issues you have, whether diagnosed or undiagnosed, these result from situations and unresolved issues. You may even believe you have moved on and 'got over' some events from the past but often this is not the case.

Here is one example:

One of my clients came to me with the shingles virus. The

skin had mostly cleared up but he was still suffering fatigue, aches and other symptoms of the virus. I know, through my work with mind-body connections, that shingles is an issue related to contact socially. This may be having contact we do not want, such as abuse, or missing someone through grief or some sort of separation.

On his first session, my client mentioned that he had lost his nan. She was not only his nan but the woman who brought him up. She was more of a mother to him. He added "but I've dealt with it now". I flagged this issue in my mind because I was fairly confident this was the cause of the shingles.

In his second session, when he was relaxed, and I asked him to advise me of an event which needed to be addressed, losing his nan came up. We were able to release the emotion and create a more positive resolution for his subconscious mind. Had he been able to release the emotion much earlier then the physical issue would not have occurred. When I saw him on his next session, he felt so much better. His energy had improved and he had turned a massive corner to creating good health.

This is a little insight into the connection between unresolved mental and emotional issues and physical well-being. Prolonged or repetitive well-being concerns, whether mental, emotional or physical, are usually messages of unresolved matters.

It is easy to disregard events from the past as the cause to current issues because you believe you have dealt with them or are over those experiences. You assume that you have somehow come to terms with the situations or you rarely think about them, if at all. Sometimes people believe they have got over an event or should be over it because it happened so many years ago. We hear that time is a healer but this is not always true. The truth is that past events very much impact the present.

The most powerful way to create change comes through working with the subconscious mind and using energy techniques to work with your body's natural meridian system. This is why I am so damn passionate about the work I do because I have witnessed such incredible changes. This resolution gives me such belief in people and their ability to change, as long as they commit to the process.

Considering the life example, I have provided, you can understand how connected the mind and body are. You may believe you have recovered from something or 'got over it' but in terms of your own internal processing and messaging system, there remains something unresolved.

The mental health issues you are dealing with are highly likely to be the result of stressful situations, whether these are events from the past, decades ago or more recent. The stress may be short term or long term.

STRESS HAS TO GO SOMEWHERE WHETHER IT AFFECTS YOU PHYSICALLY, EMOTIONALLY OR MENTALLY

The mind is exceptionally powerful, it can be your best friend or your worst enemy depending on how you use it.

My message to you is that mental health problems usually result from events which happen in life. Often these begin as a child when we are very open to suggestion and struggle to make sense of the world. If we form a negative view of ourselves as a young child, we will spend our lives reconfirming that view over and over and this will develop into our truth. It then becomes hard to break that cycle, unless we are able to gain new insight or heal the original trigger.

There are many triggers for mental health issues. To give you examples, I have listed some potential situations which may cause mental health issues and the types of response we have to them. This list is purely an example to give you an overview:

Event	**Possible response**
Being bullied	Lack confidence. Suffer anxiety.
Failing exams	Depression. Negative view of self.
Relationship struggles	Addiction in a bid to hide the negative feelings
Being made redundant	Depression and lack of self-worth
Bereavement	Emotional eating, depression
Work pressures	Insomnia. Anger outbursts.
Childhood sexual abuse	Anxiety, depression and OCD

Mental health issues can lead to secondary negative

responses. If you suffer anxiety or depression for a long time, these can then lead to insomnia, addictions, self-harm, eating disorders, fears and phobias, OCD and personality disorders. Alternatively, these issues may be initial responses to stress and trauma, which then result in anxiety or depression. There is no hard and fast rule when it comes to developing mental health issues.

Having a mental health issue does not make you weak, useless or hopeless. It means that you have unresolved issues.

Mental health problems are a response to those unresolved issues, stresses or traumas.

Your brain is in overload processing the information and trying to make sense of it. Therefore, life becomes overwhelming. However, those issues can be addressed which means you can lead a much better life. This may take some time. It will take commitment but it is possible.

I wonder what you think about your mental health challenges. How do you see yourself? Do you believe you are doing the best you can in life? Are you far too tough on yourself?

My guess is you are being much harder on yourself than you should be and you are lambasting yourself for not being able to sort your own head out. This could be because, until now, you had not considered that your mental health issues are a response to the stresses and difficulties faced in life. These could go back decades. They reflect how the mind works. However, they are not a reflection of the brilliant person you are.

Some people are more vulnerable to mental health issues

and others to physical. This is a fact of life. However, it does not matter who you are, whether you are successful, white, Asian, black, gay, non-binary, transsexual, rich, poor, beautiful, fit, single, married or anything else, mental health is not something reserved for any one segment of society. Problems can hit us at any time in our lives. It is a response to situations, that is all.

When clients come to me with any type of mental health issue, my first thought is "what has caused this?" What I do not think is "this person is flawed, hopeless, useless or bad" or any other adjectives you use to describe yourself because none of that is true.

Your mental health struggles are a reflection of something which is unresolved and requires releasing and healing.

It is important to seek out the root cause in order to achieve resolution and bring the real you back. You may not know the reason initially and that is absolutely fine as there may also be a number of causes. In therapy terms we call this peeling away the layers of an onion. Each layer represents another aspect to be released and resolved. Healing and recovery is a process. Our minds are incredible. Decades after an event has happened, we can release the stress and trauma being held in our minds and bodies and start to create a healthy state of mind.

There is more than hope, there is resolution.

Genetics and mental health issues

Reports suggest that mental health issues may be partially related to genetics. A gene is made up of segments of deoxyribonucleic acid. This is what we know as DNA. A difference in the DNA sequence is what causes a gene variant. In theory this gene variant can be a trigger for health issues.

People who have a parent with mental health issues are sometimes concerned that they will also develop similar problems. Whether we have a predisposition to any type of illness through genetics, we may never activate those genes. In effect, those genes can be turned on or off.

If we have a parent who suffers anxiety, then we may develop anxiety through 'learned behaviour'. This means we are more likely to mimic that behaviour. Therefore, this response would not necessarily be gene related.

If you have witnessed a parent struggle with depression during your childhood, being in that environment may cause mental health issues, possibly through suppressing your own emotions and feeling isolated or unsupported.

If one of your parents struggled with alcoholism throughout your childhood, this is a very unhealthy environment to be brought up in, which may have triggered mental health issues. It is not uncommon for someone brought up in such an environment to lack confidence, have low self-esteem and suffer anxiety or depression.

You could think of a genetic predisposition to a mental or physical health condition, i.e. a gene variant, as a button. That button may never be pressed. In which case the health condition never occurs. **It is only if certain factors are apparent that the button is pressed and the health issue activated. The genetic predisposition to a health issue would remain dormant if not activated.**

Therefore, although some DNA markers for mental health issues may be apparent, it is more likely that environmental factors will be the cause of mental health issues. An environmental factor is any upset in your life such as a death, changing schools or job, accident, bullying, divorce, being made redundant, dysfunctional upbringing, falling out with friends or any other stress.

We should consider that many people who have mental health conditions, probably have no predisposition to the health condition.

It is important to note that, in the same way the button can be pressed to activate the health condition, it can also be unpressed to deactivate the health condition. In terms of mental health, this would usually follow therapy. I do not include medication in this because medication hides symptoms. It does not cure. In order to keep the button unpressed and health in good order, this may also require certain environmental markers to be stable but in many cases it is possible.

To clarify what I mean by stable environmental markers. This would be minimising stressful or traumatic situations or to develop techniques for dealing with stressful situations and releasing emotions. It may also involve general well-being activities and a good work-life balance. A support network either through professionals, family or friends might also be beneficial.

5. Back to you

We have established that modern day life is more complicated than you were prepared for naturally. Some aspects of this may be difficult to change. However, it is often possible to change perception and to release some stress that goes with it.

I want you to know that whatever you are experiencing; if it has a name, such as anxiety or depression, or if it does not have a name, then you are completely justified in what you are feeling and experiencing. I have spoken to men who have questioned their experiences and whether others have the same challenges.

Men often believe they are the only one struggling in this way and therefore think they are at fault. The truth is other men are going through the same or similar experiences to you. You are not alone in the challenges you are facing. Whether you are suffering anxiety, depression or any other mental health issue, this is a response to life events which have yet to be overcome.

I can confirm, with confidence, that you are not crazy, whacky, weird (well, no more than the rest of us) or useless. You have reacted to stress of some sort and, as I have already said, it has to go somewhere. By picking up this book, you are doing something about it.

Knowing what is the root cause of the struggles you are having can pave the way to freedom. Some men know why they are feeling the way they do and others are not sure. If you are not sure, it is possible that what you are experiencing is because of several factors. It may be related to events which have happened to you over your entire lifetime.

Often men will come into my studio and tell me about something that has happened to them way back in the past and then tell me "but I have dealt with that" or "I am over it". However, during a session that memory arises because, subconsciously, it remains unresolved. It is still playing on your mind similar to a movie running over and over, reminding you of that traumatic or stressful event and causing havoc in your life.

Perhaps you do not know the root cause to the struggles you are having. This is also a common situation. This is why we are exploring many topics. Some will create that light bulb moment for you. At the very least, by reading this book, you will be asking your subconscious to reveal what is behind your struggles.

I will explain a little more about some potential reasons for mental health issues throughout this book. There will be some adjustments you can make for yourself. Other issues are best dealt with through therapy, which I will explain more about too. I will share some real-life experiences from client sessions.

Through the course of this book, you will realise there are many reasons for mental health issues and gain insight into the workings of your own mind.

6. Steps to change

Awareness

Sometimes the downturn in our mental health can happen at such a gradual rate it becomes the normal. Therefore, it can take something significant, such as the breakdown of a relationship or losing your job, to appreciate that something is wrong. The fact you are reading this book suggests to me that you recognise you need to address your mental health. Alternatively, someone has given you the book in the hope you will take some action for your own well-being. You may of course be reading this in a bid to understand others better and help them. If so, well done, that is a sensible thing to do. The more awareness we can all have towards mental health the better.

At the moment you may not know whether you have depression, anxiety or what specifically is the issue. As you progress through this book, you will gain greater insight and understand yourself better.

Acknowledgement

Sometimes we know something is not right but we put off addressing it in the hope it will go away. If you find the difficulties you are experiencing do not go away then it is time to get them addressed. Remember what you are experiencing is a symptom. This may be to do with an event you buried deep in your subconscious because you could not face it. It may be because of a series of stresses and now your health is the message which is telling you to address them. At this stage, all you need to do is acknowledge whatever it is you are experiencing and continue from there.

Talk to someone

Talking to someone will help you lift that heavy weight off your shoulders. I hope you have someone in your life who you trust and are ready to open up dialogue with. This may be to seek professional help or to explain how you feel to someone you are comfortable with. Once you talk you will feel better. You have made a proactive approach to change. If you do not have a relative, partner, friend or colleague who you can talk to, then seek out a therapist.

Look after your well-being

Well-being is significant to good mental health. There may be simple changes you can make to your well-being, which will help you create a better state of mental health.

You can be proactive by taking small steps such as listening to podcasts and watching YouTube videos on well-being, reading personal development books and finding someone to talk to. There is more information on well-being to follow.

Find out options for help

There are lots of options for help. You have a catalogue of ways to self-help through this book. This may be all that you need. You may feel that you are not in a place to help yourself and that you are best going straight to professional help. Either way, do something that will help even if you are a little sceptical.

It helps to gain knowledge of someone else's experience of a good therapist so you can get a recommendation but if this is not possible, look at the testimonials on the therapist's website.

Professional help

It may surprise you to find out what types of treatments can help. It has surprised my clients that hypnotherapy and other techniques and systems I use can create such positive change. People rarely consider hypnotherapy to help with depression but I have found it powerful. Professional help can guide you towards continued self-help for your own well-being if you need direction. For example, I may suggest to my clients to do breathing exercises, listen to one of my recordings, to read a particular book or to limit their social media.

Whether or not you seek professional help may depend on a few things:

- If you qualify for therapy or group well-being programmes through government-funded schemes
- Available finances (if going private)
- How bad you feel
- To what extent the difficulties you are feeling impact your life and those close to you
- How determined you are to feel good
- Whether you feel you can address matters yourself and are motivated to do so
- Whether you need professional guidance and support

Attend sessions with professional

If you go down the route of professional help please be consistent in attending your sessions. It is important to commit to the process. You should be asked for feedback every session. In most cases you should notice some improvement by session three or earlier. If you do feel you are not making progress then raise this with your therapist.

They may shed light on why it is taking a while for you to begin feeling the benefit of the sessions.

Don't leave all the work to the therapist

If your therapist sets you tasks to do at home, please do them. This is for your own good and will help you progress. When working with my clients, those who do additional tasks I set them at home will reap the benefits.

Continue sessions until sign off

If you seek therapeutic help then continue sessions until your therapist signs you off. Sometimes people feel a little better and stop sessions before all the underlying issues are addressed. The result of this may be a return to mental health problems. In some cases, this could be quite sudden.

This is assuming that you are making good progress with your therapist. If you are not, then you may need to find another therapist, possibly a different type of therapy. However, before you change therapist, please bear in mind my earlier comment about raising the issue if you are not making progress after three sessions.

Maintain awareness of well-being

When we are in a good place, both physically and mentally, we think less about how we feel because it is not an issue. There is no need to focus overly on your well-being once you feel better, although you should continue doing some of the activities which have led to your improvement. If you notice a decline in your mental well-being, consider what the cause might be and seek to resolve any issues which arise.

When you feel better it should be easier to notice the triggers which cause you to experience difficulties. Having this awareness can help you to make informed decisions about certain situations. For example, if work gets too busy, you may address the issue earlier than you would have done in the past or if you start to feel anxious, you may recognise the trigger and address it.

Having worked through the underlying emotional issues with one of my clients, we could then isolate one particular issue which recurred occasionally. They experienced a dissociated type of feeling when not grounded. As long as he went for some walks on the beach or used alternative methods for grounding himself, he could keep his well-being in good form.

If you find things slip you may book an appointment with your therapist so you can address the issue at an early stage and resolve it quickly. Once you build up a relationship with your therapist, it can be so much easier to have a top-up session because the initial trepidation has gone and you have built up a trusting relationship.

7. Opening up to someone close

When any member of a family has mental health issues, there is a strain experienced by everyone in the family. This is an excellent reason to find an outlet for your emotions and take some action so you can enjoy life more.

Men will often bottle up their negative thoughts and feelings because they do not want to worry their family or friends or cause any stress in what probably is already a busy life. However, if you fail to address what you are worrying about or feeling, it will most likely get worse and become a larger issue to deal with. Mental health problems rarely go away without some intervention, whether that is making some changes for yourself or seeking professional help.

Mental health struggles may cause you to have a short temper, feel frustrated and get angry more easily. In extreme cases you could become violent. Although this is not the person you are. This is the person who is struggling and is caught up in emotions, not knowing how to release them in a healthy way.

If you notice your temper is short, it is likely to be those closest to you who are at the receiving end. This may cause arguments and unease within the household. If you have a short fuse, please talk about it so that your partner, friends or family understand the anger is not personal towards them. Then you can discuss how to address the issue. Having the support of someone, whether it is your partner, a friend or family member is incredibly beneficial.

At the other end of the emotional spectrum are issues such as anxiety and depression. You might flip between a variety of feelings and emotions. Often friends and family are keen to help and support you but are not sure how to broach the subject and so procrastinate. This results in the status quo.

For a partner or family, these can be tricky times because they want to help you. They want you to feel better and have a wonderful life but they can often feel helpless themselves. Therefore, talking is essential. For them to gain insight into what you are feeling and experiencing can help to pave the way to seeking the right help for you. It is amazing what a weight it can be off your shoulders when you open up the communication. You might just be surprised at how much support there is for you.

You could write a letter to explain what you are feeling and the thoughts you are having. Instead, you may record a voice message to the person you decide to confide in. If you are more artistic, create a drawing or painting which shows what is happening or how it feels inside your mind. Write a poem or song. There are different ways to express those emotions and feelings.

It is not always easy to articulate exactly what you are feeling in words but that is fine. You can say "I know I am not 100%. Something feels wrong but I cannot tell you what." Sometimes it is difficult to know if you are depressed or anxious or if you are experiencing something else. You do not need to diagnose the issue. Just put your hand up and ask for help.

I have prepared a communication form in the appendix to help you with this. You could either hand it to your chosen confidante or use it as the basis for a chat with them. If you do not have a partner, you can use this document with another family member, colleague, therapist or friend but please do have that conversation.

Section 1

Understanding yourself and where things start to go wrong

Gaining insight into the reasons why you are struggling, is the first step to empowerment and change.

8. What you believe is important

If you have read any of my other books, you will know how relevant our own personal beliefs are to how we live our lives. What we believe is important. However, what we believe is not always the truth.

Look into your internal dialogue, the things you are telling yourself. For example, are you telling yourself:

"I'm hopeless"
"I'm rubbish"
"I'm a disaster"

Most people who experience mental health issues will have a negative internal dialogue about themselves based on their personal belief system.

If our mind was a computer then our beliefs are our operating system. As long as we believe we are awesome, capable, brilliant, great company, can achieve anything and a good person then chances are we will breeze through life and not get upset by much. Should someone be negative towards us or we make a mistake, then we can keep it in perspective and appreciate that it does not define the person we are. However, the reality of life can be quite different to this.

Let us have a look at where some of your beliefs might have come from. Life experiences are fundamental in forming our beliefs:

Bullying	Seeing others doing well
Mistakes	Overprotective parent

News	Development issues
Dyslexia	A sibling being more successful
Religion	Negative & critical comments
Media	Perceived Failure
Accident	Parent with struggles
Injury	Struggling at school
Abuse	Failing an exam
Illness	Social media
Bereavement	Negative behaviour from others

In stress or trauma, we will experience an emotion which could be anything from disgust to fear. At that time, we usually form a belief linked to our perception of that event. Beliefs are personal and varied. Common types of beliefs are:

"I'm not good enough"
"I'm all alone in this world"
"I need to show I'm strong"
"It is important for people to like me"

You may not be aware of your beliefs consciously. However, they are locked into your subconscious mind. As a result of those beliefs, you will then create a response, usually in the form of habits or behaviours.

Put simply, an event which has an emotional trigger will usually cause us to form beliefs, especially at a young age. Those beliefs can change the way we view ourselves, others and the world at large. They also impact how we deal with future situations and are largely responsible for the habits we form. Usually, those habits and behaviours are created to protect or soothe ourselves, although sometimes might be to hurt or punish ourselves.

**Event/Trauma
(Emotion/Reaction)**

↓

Belief

↓

**Response:
Future Habit/Behaviour**

A single event can change your view of yourself, other people or the world. At the time of the event, your perception closed down, your knowledge, skills and wisdom could not be accessed. You are in the fight, flight or freeze response. This is your natural protective mechanism.

When you review those events at a later date, your initial reaction and belief formed at the time may appear dramatic or nonsensical. However, in stress and trauma, we do not have the balance of logical thought and the ability to assess every aspect of the situation. It is as if we are in a tunnel and only have our natural survival response to help us.

Let us look more specifically at types of events which change our view of ourselves, others and the world.

Childhood events

Childhood is significant in creating our belief system. We

form most of our beliefs before we are seven years old. This becomes a problem because, as a young child, we do not have the ability to form a balanced perspective on many situations. We are unable to recognise or access all of our resources in terms of skills, talents, wisdom and understanding at such a young age. We form a view of the situation in a particular moment based on our limited knowledge and life experience. This can cause us to hold on to unhelpful and negative beliefs.

We live in a world with social media and 24/7 news. This means children are much more aware nowadays of everything happening in the world. However, they do not have the capacity to understand situations fully and balance the good and bad news. This results in many irrational fears and anxieties.

Later, I talk about childhood abuse, which can certainly result in unhelpful beliefs. However, many other situations can lead to a belief system which causes us to doubt ourselves, holds us back in life or creates irrational fear.

Now follows some examples of the types of situations which lead to creating an understandably challenging belief system.

Event	**Belief**
You hear about a plane crash and your school friends are talking about all the people on the plane dying	You believe that flying is dangerous.

You struggle academically at school	You believe you are stupid and won't amount to much.
You witness your dad hit your mum (or vice versa)	You believe you are weak for not doing anything to protect your mum.
You are bullied	You believe you are weird or unpopular.
Your mum and dad split up	You believe you must have done something wrong to cause this and are therefore are a bad person.
A parent or sibling frequently tells you that you are useless	You believe you are useless.

There are many beliefs we can form, which become the foundation for how we function in life. Let us now look at how these beliefs may cause someone to behave:

Belief	**Response/Behaviour**
Flying is dangerous	Refuse to fly or become extremely anxious at the thought of flying.
I am stupid	Avoid studying and say little in social gatherings because you do not believe you have anything of worth to contribute

I am weak	Self-loathe. Become withdrawn. Fear confrontation.
I am weird	Become withdrawn. Uneasy with social interaction of any sort.
I'm a bad person	Self-loathe. Self-sabotage. Stop yourself enjoying life or achieving.
I am useless	Never strive for achievement. Keep yourself constrained to simple tasks. Limit ambitions.

There are many ways our beliefs can impact our lives. When we carry a negative view of ourselves, this can limit our enjoyment of life, our ambition and motivation. This is where the negativity festers and turns into a range of long-term issues such as anxiety, depression, addiction, emotional eating, self-harm or obsessive-compulsive behaviour. If we can understand our belief system better then we can start to change the internal programming.

When a client explains what they are experiencing, such as depression or anxiety, my first thought is "where has this come from?" Problems occur for a reason. They do not just happen. The reason may not be obvious but will usually rise to the surface. Do not dismiss anything as a possible root cause or contributor to the challenges you are facing because it seems too insignificant, too long ago or irrelevant. If it rises to the surface, my experience tells me it is for a reason. That reason is that it is relevant and needs to be addressed.

What do you believe?

Below is a list of possible beliefs you may hold, which could have a relevance to your mental and emotional well-being. Using the list below note how relevant you feel they are to you, in your life currently, in percentage terms. Alternatively use a scale of 0-10 if you prefer.

You may feel some are completely irrelevant. In which case mark as zero, others may be completely relevant, therefore these would be around the 100% mark. Of course, others may be anywhere else on the scale. The trick is to do this quickly and go with the first number that pops into your head. In the weeks or months ahead, you can repeat this exercise to see how your beliefs have changed, as you drop the issues which have been holding you back.

Belief	**Score %**
I'm not good enough	
I'm hopeless	
I feel isolated/abandoned	
No-one listens to me	
I'm not confident enough	
I'm not clever enough	
I'm unforgivable	
I'm flawed/something is wrong with me	
I'll get things wrong/I'm useless	

I'm unlovable	
People are out to get me	
I'm insignificant	
People take advantage of me	
I'm weak	
People judge me	
I must show others I'm strong	
Something bad will happen	

I have included a couple of blank boxes in case you are aware of any other key beliefs you hold which are limiting you.

If you notice that you tend to run through the same negative thoughts, or respond to situations with a recurring negative comment about yourself, then add that to the list. In any event, the above list gives you a good basis to understand yourself better.

The high scores are an indication of a belief which has a strong influence on how you see yourself or other aspects of life. This will have an impact on your mental and emotional well-being. These scores reflect your own reality but not 'the reality'. They have set the programme for how you live your life and create restrictions. Often those restrictions stop you enjoying life to the full. They stop you having a positive opinion of yourself and reaching your full potential.

These negative beliefs are formed based on one or more experience in your life. They are part of a snapshot of your life. You hold that belief as if it were locked into you. Through this locked-in belief, you missed an opportunity to recognise and appreciate so many wonderful things about yourself and life.

In my experience, people are far more awesome than they realise. They are more capable than they believe and they have wonderful skills, talents and personality traits which they fail to recognise.

Need to be strong

Some people see mental health issues as some kind of weakness. I hope you are beginning to appreciate that they are more likely a sign of being strong for too long and having put up with significant stress or trauma. Mental health issues are experienced by amazing people who have suffered difficulties.

Commonly as a boy, you may have been told by your father or another adult that you need to be tough or act like a man. Perhaps this was a time when you were crying. By being told this, you were denied your emotions. This is not a criticism of your father or whoever said it because this is what they believed and were probably told themselves. This is what people used to think was the case. However, we are living in a changing and more diverse world where we acknowledge, accept and express emotions more freely.

You should never be denied your feelings. There is absolutely no weakness in showing your emotions. When we cry, we are releasing emotions, which is a good thing. It is far better to express how we feel than to lock those emotions in.

If we suppress emotions, they will reveal themselves at a later date and usually in an unhealthy way.

A suppressed emotion becomes troublesome. It is important to establish that emotions are good. They are a sign of our state of being. What we call negative emotions, such as sadness, anger or frustration, are a sign that something that is happening or has happened does not sit well with us. Emotions are information. They are part of us. They are part of you. Therefore, it is important to understand emotions and to develop more helpful ways of dealing with them.

As an adult you may still believe you need to be the strong one in your relationship. People may rely on you. You should be able to cope. To let out emotions does not suggest that you cannot cope. Quite the contrary. It is the healthy way to be. At times in life, we all go through challenges. During those times we need support. We need to speak and express how we feel freely without fear of judgement.

The same is true of any problems or worries you have. You will feel a great release when you talk those through. I am sure you know the saying "a problem shared is a problem halved". This is because just by saying whatever is bothering you out loud, you have released some of the stress you were holding in. Talking through your problems can take the sting away, lessening the overall impact they have on you. Bringing in support, guidance and new perspectives can be a great help.

Sometimes, my clients will tell me of an event, situation or worry. This may be something they have held onto for years and never told another person. After they have told me they feel so much better. It can feel as if a heavy weight has been lifted off their shoulders.

Holding on to stressful information or a trauma for years can take its toll physically, mentally and emotionally. Do not underestimate the possible impact of this on you. Find a confidante who you feel safe to talk to. This might be a friend you have known for years, your partner, a colleague, your massage therapist, personal trainer or a therapist.

9. When to seek help

As a generalisation, men are not very good at seeking help. The result of this is that life can become intolerable before help is sought. Whether the trigger be losing your job, insomnia, relationship problems, friendship fall-outs, addiction, self-harm, panic attacks, anxiety, depression or any other issue. Often, if you seek help at an early stage, matters can be dealt with very swiftly.

As a hypnotherapist, I often find myself being the last resort for people. This is mainly because people do not understand hypnotherapy and sometimes because of the nonsense they see on television with stage-style hypnosis, which is very different to the therapeutic approach.

By the time many clients come to me they have explored all other avenues, including the doctor, medication, counselling, cognitive behaviour therapy (CBT), other forms of holistic treatments and sometimes even other hypnotherapists. My job is often tougher because, by this stage, I have in front of me a person who is at the end of their tether and has little, if any, belief that they can recover.

However, with commitment, we do turn things around. This happens at different speeds for different people for a number of reasons:

- The background and depth of issues to be resolved.
- The impact of the background issues on their mental, emotional and physical well-being.
- Current stresses in their life.
- Commitment to sessions.
- Commitment to doing any out of session suggestions,

such as listening to MP3s or other actions for well-being.

Here are a few areas to be aware of. If you find that you are impacted by any of the following, then I suggest seeking help. I have included an approximate time frame to give you guidance but, if in any doubt whatsoever, seek immediate advice or help.

- Feelings of desperation or suicide - seek help immediately. Do not delay!
- Turning to substances or other unhealthy behaviour to switch your mind off, e.g. alcohol, gambling or porn. Seek help immediately.
- Develop anger issues or violence. Seek help immediately.
- Struggle to get up in the morning for more than 5 days.
- Negative thoughts or feelings towards yourself for more than 5 days.
- Sleep is impacted for more than 7 days.
- Constant or frequent worrying for more than 7 days.
- Unusual physical feelings in your body for more than 7 days. These could be anything but common feelings are butterflies or tightness in the stomach, chest or throat.
- Lack motivation or energy for more than 7 days.

You may be surprised at how quickly I am suggesting seeking help. This is because if you deal with matters sooner rather than later, it is possible to return to good mental health again in a matter of weeks, possibly sooner. That help may be of a friend, colleague or family member initially. This saves you struggling for months, years or decades as some men do.

10. Should, could, would

Assuming you are not doing well enough at life can affect your mindset. Those who experience mental health issues often compare themselves to others and believe everyone else is doing better in all areas of life. They also run over and over those situations which should have gone better. They recall situations when they let others down or the events which they are not proud of and run them over and over in their mind.

You tell yourself:

"I **should** be doing better than I am."
"I **could** have got that promotion if I was more assertive".
"I **would** own my own house if I had knuckled down years ago".

I recall speaking to someone who was a successful sports person and had recently started up his own business. Despite his successes, he made a flippant comment to me that he was "failing at life". To everyone else this guy had it all, but underneath there were cracks and he believed he was not doing well enough.

Another guy said to me, "if you look at my social media accounts, you would assume I am happy and confident. The truth is, I am struggling". This person lacked confidence and felt depressed. However, to the rest of the world he was living the dream in a career he loved.

One of my clients was chastising himself for one shoplifting incident that happened when he was 10-years-old. He had carried negative feelings about himself because of this event for approximately 40 years. He believed he was a terrible person. At 50-years-old he had not yet put the event into perspective because of his deeply held belief that the incident meant he was a bad person.

Another client had cheated in a sporting event. At the time he was at a low point in life but, in his words, he told me how cheating had made him feel "it broke me".

One thing which is so hard about these types of issues and events is that we struggle to let them go. We want to bury them in the hope they go away but they remain unresolved and carry a strong emotional charge which you try to suppress. You may feel so bad about something you did many years ago that you could not tell the person closest to you because of the shame you continue to feel.

If you formed a negative belief about yourself because of a specific event, you would have held that inside of you and kept it to yourself. It hurt you over and over again. This would have left you unable to gain a fair perspective of the event or yourself because your viewpoint was narrow and fixed.

In life we all do things we are not proud of. However, at the time and in that situation, we were possibly naïve, unhappy, desperate, trying to fit in with others, striving to feel more powerful, had a low regard for ourselves or did not understand fully or consider the impact of our actions. Sometimes we do things which are illogical and out of character given the benefit of hindsight. Good people do silly or bad things but they are not bad people.

It serves no purpose to hold the past against yourself. If you do anything, use the past as a springboard to becoming a

Stresses of Modern Man

better version of yourself. Do something for the community, do a good deed or help someone out. These are far better ways to even things up than to chastise yourself.

The important point to consider is whether you would do that same action now. If the answer is "no", you are not that same person. You have learned, and that is a great positive. Give yourself a pat on the back for bringing understanding into that situation. If you believe you owe an apology, make the apology. You will feel better and it allows you to wipe the slate clean.

The fact that you feel bad says that you have changed. It tells me you are an honourable person and have learned the lesson. However, holding onto bad feelings about yourself is a continuous punishment which serves no purpose. There is no benefit to anyone if you continue to feel bad about the past.

Put into perspective, the man who shoplifted at age 10 spent 40 years believing he was a terrible person because of that one act. Let's face it, you get less for committing murder.

Believing that you have not lived up to expectation is a common feeling amongst men. One client of mine, I will call Steve, had set himself some life goals. He planned to travel the world and buy a house before he became 30 years old. Neither of which happened, causing him to believe he had failed in life.

Interestingly, Steve did not want to travel. It was just something he felt he should tick off because many of his peers were travelling in their twenties. If something does not suit us, we need not follow others just to tick that box. Life is for having the experiences you want and from which you will thrive. You are wonderfully unique. It is important that you do what feels right for you.

At the time Steve came to see me he held a low opinion of himself because of his preconceived idea of how he should be and the life he was leading. What he had failed to do was to recognise how amazing he was. He is one of the nicest men I have ever met and an absolute pleasure to work with. However, he had spent his time chastising himself for not living up to his own expectations of the life he should live. Life is not that straightforward though.

Some situations throw us off course. These could be a dysfunctional childhood, challenges at school, difficult friendship groups, relationship issues, grief, making mistakes that we cannot get over, job problems, ill health and traumas. We spend life negotiating our way through challenges and fail to register how well we are doing.

When anyone is pushed too far, the cracks will appear. Often those cracks open up slowly. Perhaps a dreadful night's sleep or a few digestive issues. Negative thoughts may creep in. This gradual decline continues until one day you realise you have lost all control of how you are feeling. This is, without doubt, distressing and scary.

Praise yourself sometimes. Initially this is probably a hard thing to do, but I assure you that you are doing great, given whatever struggles and challenges you have dealt with to this point in time. The very fact you are reading this book tells me you want to make changes. This is positive.

I see clients every day in my studio who have been to hell and back and I sometimes think to myself "wow, how are you even breathing" or "how are you functioning", "how have you done so well". These are incredible people and they are no different to you. You could easily be one of these people and, just as they do, fail to register how brilliantly you have done in life. Give yourself a break. Whatever you believe you should have done, either it is not too late or it was never meant to be. You are here now, doing your best.

Through addressing the underlying issues and helping Steve tap into new perspectives, he was feeling so much better in himself. He then put in place plans to buy a property. He felt fantastic about this. When he came for his last session with me, the wheels were set in motion for purchasing a property later that year.

Life is about decisions. One decision may affect another part of life. It is important to set priorities which are important to you and not to fit in or please others at the detriment of your well-being or happiness.

A wonderful thing about getting older is you have life experiences to call upon and I could explain to Steve that being 30 is not a brick wall. There is plenty you can achieve after 30. I changed career twice, once at 37 and once at 40. If I can make changes in my mid-life so can you. People run marathons in their nineties. There is no age limit on achieving success.

There may be many things about today's life that cause more stress but we also have more opportunities nowadays. Sometimes we ignore the opportunities available and disregard the power we hold to change our lives. We can make changes any time. There is no need to be stuck in a bad or unsuitable relationship, career or lifestyle. We are not doomed to be miserable forever. Let go of self-judgement and look towards a brighter future, knowing you can make changes happen.

Those challenging times are snapshots of life. They do not define the person you are or have the last say in what you can achieve. Everyone struggles in life at some point. Even those who appear to have everything, as if good things fall into their lap, have struggles of their own. We all make mistakes, or would change at least one aspect of our life if we could. Through my work, I have realised that, we are not very different from each other. The key difference is our perception. Our impression of ourselves, others and life experiences is critical. I hope that through this book, you will gain fresh perspectives.

We pass through these tough periods in life. How quickly we pass through them depends on us. Are you motivated for change and willing to do what is necessary?

Living in the past does not serve you in the present or the future. There is so much life to enjoy ahead of you. You can create opportunities, learn a new skill, or flourish in a fulfilling career, you can do many things with focus, commitment and dedication. Now is the right time to consider the life you want and take some steps towards fulfilling your desires.

11. Lack of fulfilment

Many people feel unfulfilled in life. It saddens me that so many people wake up on a Monday morning and want it to be Friday evening as soon as possible. People wish away over 70% of their week. For some people work is a significant reason they are unfulfilled. Other reasons may be related to relationships, financial challenges, family issues, negative feelings about themselves and underachievement.

Any type of conflict can potentially become destructive. Believing you are not fulfilling your role as a partner, husband, son, dad or colleague. Being dissatisfied in any area of your life. Thinking you are not good enough. These are common areas of conflict.

With unfulfillment often comes feelings of hopelessness or helplessness. You believe life controls you and you have no say in how things pan out. You may believe you are a victim of the hand you were dealt. Functioning day-to-day is a chore. These are feelings linked with depression.

This will probably be because of your life experiences, including the stressful experiences you have been through and what you may be going through now.

I have witnessed many people turn this around, which results in making empowering decisions for themselves. This is due to a change in their belief system. They believe more in themselves; they gain more confidence and realise they have a greater say in how they live their life. Sometimes this involves big decisions such as ending an unhealthy relationship, changing career, travelling, moving house or asking for a promotion.

At times, situations in life can be challenging to downright awful. Some people unfortunately experience more than their fair share of stressful or traumatic events. We may not be able to change the past but we are the creators of our future and have a say in what happens in our lives.

To create the life we want, we must know what we desire. Many people do not have a clue as to what that may be, however they know they do not want the life they currently have. It is therefore important to consider how you would like your life to be. We all want to win the lottery, well most of us do. I would be the last person to say that is not possible but only a small percentage of participants win a big prize. However, there are changes we can make, even if tough decisions are needed.

Take a moment to consider what you would like your life to be like. What would it be like to wake up in the morning, feeling content, energised and ready for the day ahead? Those of us lucky enough to have a career we are fulfilled by gain great satisfaction from work. What is the career you want? Perhaps you already have that or you may need to gain some qualifications. If so, set the wheels in motion to achieve those qualifications. What gives you joy? What are you passionate about? Where do you want to live? What do you want family life to be like?

To create fulfilment, joy and happiness, we must first know what we desire. Once we know that, we can work towards it.

The life we desire does not come all at once and it may not end up perfect but there will be changes you can make right now to create a life more in line with how you want to live. Whatever your current situation is the starting point to that process. Consider the future you want and then fill in the gaps to reach that future. You can take it one step at a time.

12. The male introvert

Social contact is a basic human need. However, if there was a scale of desire for social contact across the board, this would vary considerably. Some people need continuous human connection, whereas others can go days, even weeks, without any and feel absolutely fine. There is no one-size-fits-all when it comes to our need for human connection.

In reality, many of us cross the border between introvert and extrovert. It was psychologist, Carl Jung, who identified the difference between introverts and extroverts back in the 1960s when he separated each type by how they were re-energised. Introverts need time alone to boost their energy, which is drained by interaction with others. Extroverts, on the other hand, are boosted by the company of others. We can be a mix of the two. There is no wrong or right when it comes to introverts and extroverts.

It is challenging being a male introvert, especially as a youngster through to mid-thirties. Our stereotypical male is fired up on testosterone, wants to play with Lego at any age, likes football, cricket and motorsport, loves a beer, is confident with the ladies and loves a night out with the lads.

An introvert finds the company of others tiring. Big groups would be draining. Introverts are often more comfortable in the company of very small groups or on a one-to-one basis. They will also need time to themselves to reboot their energy.

Introverts are not skilled conversationalists, unless they are talking about a subject they are interested in. They find small-talk rather tedious.

Life as an introvert may be more in line with the following:

- Most relaxed and happy in their own company
- Prefers one-to-one or small group interaction
- In the right company, will talk about their passions
- Disinterested in small talk
- Needs time on their own to re-energise
- Not a brilliant talker
- Home is usually your safe place
- Going out is a massive chore
- Often prefers animals to humans
- Can be socially awkward
- May be more prone to depression
- Usually more comfortable chatting over text, apps or social media.
- May avoid people they know when out and about so they are not required to get into conversation. This is not out of rudeness but a feeling of dread and unconscious knowledge that the effort of doing so would drain their energy.
- Let phone calls go to voicemail. Especially unexpected calls.
- Often excellent listeners
- Self-sufficient
- Highly focused on their interests
- Can be very conscientious
- Trustworthy
- Committed to their goals
- Often deep thinkers
- They prefer limited but quality interaction
- Are likely to have just a few close friends
- Happy doing tasks or hobbies on their own.

You may not have considered yourself as an introvert but

wondered why you are not 'one of the lads'. If you relate to many of the above, you are likely to be in that awesome introvert personality category.

Introverts will often experience social anxiety particularly in large groups. Some introverts will drink alcohol in a bid to lessen their inhibitions when on a night out.

We are in a constantly evolving world, which is more accepting of our differences. This should make being an introvert more acceptable and better understood no matter what gender we are. Introvert or extrovert - neither is better than the other. Those of us who are introverts, let's be proud of our social type. Tell others you do not enjoy big social occasions and explain to them what being an introvert entails. Some people just require educating to help them understand. The more comfortable you are of being an introvert (if you are one), the less others will be able to criticise you or your behaviour.

You may find you connect with other introverts by talking about it. This can help you build friendships with people who experience life in a similar way to you. I have many friends who are introverts and the good thing is we never put pressure on each other to connect. We do not judge each other and we are comfortable in our own skin when we do meet up. Introverts are now better understood and acknowledged more than ever before but further education is needed in some areas.

Now we live in a computer age, many men are using social media and gaming as a way of human connection. This means they can do it on their terms and to their own time scale. Whilst this is comfortable and easy, some level of actual human contact is healthy. It is a positive thing to talk about your passions and to be in the company of people you can laugh with and have great rapport with. In the right circumstances, this can energise you and boost your mood.

It can still be challenging to make those connections which suit you. Sometimes male introverts find it easier connecting with females, as they can find their energy less draining. You might achieve your human connection through a sport or a hobby.

We can be a mostly introvert but a little extrovert or vice versa. I have always been an introvert, happy in my own company and quite a deep thinker. However, I have my extrovert moments. Throughout the years I have become more of an introvert and found benefit in having only a few friendships with limited social interaction. Keeping life uncomplicated has been noticeably beneficial for my well-being. If it feels good for you, then it is right for you but try not to be a complete hermit.

Being an introvert is not a slight on your personality. It is a part of your personality. If others are not accepting of this, it is their problem. It is unhealthy to act in a way which does not fit who you are in order to please others or not to be singled out as different. You need not conform to any stereotypical male from the dark ages.

Society has moved on considerably in the past century as we are more accepting of our differences. Often the thing we fear is judgement of others. However, if anyone is not accepting of introverts, they need a reality check because the world is full of them.

If you are comfortable with the person you are then others

will pick up on that and are less likely to make unnecessary or foolish comments. In any event, if they do comment in a negative way, it suggests a level of ignorance or quite possibly insecurity on their part.

My message is that it is fine to be an introvert. Do what feels right for you. You need not change this aspect of yourself. Introverts are a brilliant breed and hold many fantastic personality traits. If you are an introvert, embrace it.

13. Socialising

One of my clients, I shall call Jim, was telling me he was going out with his mates and was not looking forward to it because he did not want a late night. This was creating anxiety. He expected the event would finish in the early hours of the following day. Jim did not want to drink much alcohol either.

He was experiencing a weight of expectation that he had to stay out late and drink a fair bit of alcohol because this is what the lads would expect. This situation, and other similar situations, can cause anxiety. You want to do one thing and feel pressured to do something else, in order that you are considered 'one of the lads', but who is putting the pressure on you? The pressure is usually of our own making.

I explained to Jim that it is absolutely fine for him to decide what is best for him. If he did not want to drink at all, that is his right. If he wanted to leave at a certain time, he was within his right to do so. As a society we develop a view of social etiquette but that does not suit everyone. I talk to many people who tell me they 'have' to go out and are dreading it. However, in reality, they do not 'have' to go out at all. They have put the pressure on themselves. We need to move away from an old-fashioned view of what being sociable entails.

I told Jim that when I go out with my husband, who is more sociable than I am, I will leave before him. I also do not drink alcohol. As long as I am comfortable with these decisions all is well. It does not matter what others think because it is not their business. They have no right to tell me what to do. I want to be fresh the next morning to go out on my bike or do some writing. This will only happen if I have a reasonably early night.

If someone is putting peer pressure on you to do something, they are in the wrong. Do not be swayed and pressurised if a situation does not sit well with you. Do what is right for you.

When I saw Jim for the next session, he was thrilled because he had left the event at 11 pm and only had a pint or two. This also meant he had a much better day the following day than he would have had if he had stayed out late. In discussing the situation with me beforehand, he had realised how much alcohol he drank and what time he left were his business and his decisions to make. He released the burden of expectation he had been putting on himself. He let that go and did was what right for him and everything was fine.

Sometimes we give too much of our own power away to others for fear of retribution. However, if someone has a problem with a decision you make for your own well-being, it is their problem, not yours. Please do not take on pressure from others. By making a stance the first time, you lay the foundation for people to realise that they cannot sway you from what you want to do for your own good. You are no less of a man for not staying out with the lads or not drinking alcohol.

Doing what is right for you is not about selfishness. It is self-preservation. When we want to do one thing but feel forced to do something else, we are incongruent. There is a conflict. Initially this might create a feeling or short disturbance such as a tightening in your digestive area or throat. You might feel frustrated or a little anxious. If this continues long term the effect on us is greater. This would result in longer term health issues which could be physical, emotional or mental or a combination of these.

It is important to do what feels right to you in order to preserve your well-being. Once people start to take charge of their lives, they feel more empowered and are naturally happier.

This realisation gave Jim a feeling of freedom. He felt more in control of his life. Sometimes you need someone else to give you permission to make the right decisions for you. I am giving you that permission right now. Do what is right for you.

14. Confidence

Lack of confidence can have a strong influence on your mental well-being. People lack confidence for a variety of reasons. I will outline some viable reasons in this chapter. Once again, these are based on my client sessions and experiences. As I explain in my book, The Power of Confidence, it is unlikely that you were born with a lack of confidence. This usually happens because of experiences in life. There can be many factors to this. Upbringing has a significant part to play in this, especially if it was an abusive environment where fear was created.

Here are some reasons for lacking confidence. You may also recognise a link between these events and the beliefs you hold.

Education system

We will never achieve an education system that works for everybody. That is just never going to happen. However, if you are someone who has struggled in the schooling structure, this will have affected your confidence. Examples of experiences which affect us in this way are getting low grades, struggling to understand lessons or being overwhelmed with homework. Some youngsters feel trapped in a system which does not understand them. It is a structure which suggests that there are different levels of clever. However, intelligence is not that straightforward and comes in many forms.

For many, the schooling system leaves you feeling useless, incapable and stupid. It stops you believing in yourself and causes you to build limitations to what you can truly achieve.

There are many people who have achieved amazing things despite struggling at school. Some people have set up businesses and are millionaires or even billionaires. This goes to show that how successful we are at school is not necessarily a reflection of our abilities and intelligence. It is certainly not a precursor to every type of success in life.

For some of us trying to fit into school life is akin to trying to fit a square peg into a round hole. Unfortunately, things do not always fit. Let's face it, there are over 7 billion people in the world and over 66 million people in the UK. We are unique individuals, every one of us. We may have some similarities but we approach many things in our own way. Some of us are more capable with our hands, some more mathematical, others more athletic and others more musical or theatrical and yet we are trying to use one system to educate everyone. This is why the education system is not a positive experience for many and is not the only way to define someone's intelligence, capabilities and ability to succeed.

If you struggled at school, all that tells me is that the system was not right for you. It should not limit what you can do. Once out of the education system, you can do things your way. You can focus on the subjects and interests you are passionate about. I always believe when we are passionate about something, we will thrive.

You may have had a teacher tell you that you would not amount to much. They were wrong. They would have no idea what you could achieve because they failed to understand you. I do not blame teachers for the errors of the system. However, sometimes they lack understanding and act in a way which causes long-term damage. Some may need to be re-educated to understand how to deal with youngsters who struggle in a structure which is unsuitable for them.

Only recently a teacher was keeping a young boy in during his breaks and lunch time to finish his work because he was struggling. However, this was causing him to develop obsessive-compulsive disorder (OCD) behaviour. The boy was trying, albeit it unconsciously or unwittingly, to create some control and 'achieve' something because, the response from the teacher led him to believe he was not achieving at school. The OCD behaviour, through setting himself tasks, enabled him to achieve. These tasks were, however, inappropriate and were impacting his family unit. This is a good example of how mental health issues can develop at a very young age.

There are so many subjects in school where I learned nothing of use. What I wish for is a different style of schooling, whereby everybody can fulfil their potential. This may be where there is a university-style of teaching at a younger age, although not living in. This may involve different styles of teaching and for some who are more practically-minded, a more appropriate approach. Also enabling youngsters to explore more options and being able to pursue their strengths and passions. This is how we thrive.

Never allow yourself to be defined by any system or what others tell you. Follow your interests and passions and you will do great.

Bullying

Bullying can happen at any age and many people will experience some level of bullying in their life. If you were bullied as a youngster you may be more vulnerable to being bullied in later life because your confidence is already low.

Bullies seek out the vulnerable. They do not pick on someone they believe can stand up for themselves. They will often seek out a person who appears different. This may be someone who is quiet, unconventional looking, has an unusual walk or personality trait.

In most cases, when you stand up to bullies, they back down. This was my experience at school. At senior school I stood up to our year bully and she soon backed down. I then defended my friends when she tried to pick on them. I developed a kind of invisible coat of armour where I would pretend I was not scared of bullies. Through repeatedly standing up to bullies, this invisible coat of armour became easy to access throughout life whenever I needed it.

Bullying does not just happen in school. It can happen at home with a parent, guardian, partner or sibling. Bullying can occur in the workplace, in a social club or amongst a so-called friendship group. There is no limit to where bullying can take place.

At school, bullying is usually very personal. Perhaps you were called names. There can also be physical elements to bullying. Whatever the bully said to you was not the truth. It was their way of looking more powerful. It may have been that they were wanting to be popular so the way they went about it was to appear bigger and stronger and develop a cluster of friends who were their sheep. This creates a pack mentality.

There is also covert bullying. At school this might be leaving someone out deliberately. It can be ignoring them too. This can happen in adulthood too, even with men. Individually some covert bullying behaviour may not appear to be that big a deal but added together, it is clearly nasty. Again, it can be leaving someone out, whether that is from a conversation, making a drink for everyone else but not them or telling everyone a joke but not including them. With the latter, it could make you think they are laughing at you which is often what the bully is trying to achieve.

Bullying with guys can also appear more as bravado. Men, more than women, may play practical jokes. They may call you a derogatory name. Once again, if this continues and is more than a one-off, it is bullying. If this is happening to you, then I suggest you put them straight that you do not appreciate their behaviour. Maybe they do not realise the repercussions of their actions and never intended to hurt you. If this is happening in the workplace then speak to someone. If you get no help, write them a letter so there is a record of the communication.

Bullying is not something anyone should put up with. If the person doing the bullying is ignorant of the impact of their actions then find a way to let them know that their behaviour is causing you difficulties. If in doubt speak to a friend about the situation to gain their take on it. Know that you deserve to be treated well and there is no excuse for mistreating someone.

Bullying can cause many types of mental health issues including anxiety, depression and OCD. It can leave people lacking self-belief and confidence. It can rip out your self-worth. You may fear public speaking or being the centre of attention. You might dread change and never put yourself forward for anything, as well as telling yourself you cannot do certain things. Bullying can have a severe detrimental impact on people throughout their lives.

Bullying is a big subject. It comes in many forms. It can happen at any time in your life. If you wish to look more into this subject, I talk in more detail on bullying in my book, T*he Energy of Anxiety.*

Different Interests

Only recently a young boy came to me as he was experiencing a few emotional issues. He was telling me how he did not want to play with the other boys at break time because they played football and he did not like the game. At a young age it is especially challenging if your interests are different to the majority because this can cause you to feel isolated. You want friends but you do not enjoy what the others are doing.

During school, there is no straightforward answer to this. It depends a lot on each individual's personality. Some will join in just to be part of the group, even if they are not keen on the activity. Others may find a friend who shares the same interests and are happy to spend some break times away from the primary group.

I recall at school playing hockey with one of my best friends. The other friend was less interested but she used to come along to matches and cut up the oranges for half-time. Seeking other ways to be involved can help someone to feel included.

As adults we have more say in what we take part in. It is important to be comfortable with the person you are and your own interests. Do not hide behind those interests. Embrace them. Having different interests to the average person is brilliant. I love to hear of people's hobbies, especially if unusual. Embrace any differences you have.

We cannot be what we are not. I always encourage people to pursue their passions. Be wonderfully unique you. Pursue whatever fills you with joy, happiness and fulfilment.

For the record, it does not matter how good we are at our hobbies. I have known people apologise when talking about a hobby because they are not very good. It does not matter how good you are at it. The purpose of hobbies is to create pleasure. Never apologise for being below average at anything. How good you are is not relevant. The fun, peace or satisfaction you achieve is far more important than rating your abilities.

Dysfunctional upbringing

If family life was dysfunctional or out of the normal, then this can cause you to lack confidence.

Childhood abuse can have a significant impact on confidence levels throughout life. The impact does not just go away once you grow up and leave home. Those internal scars stay with you but can be released with help.

Other types of dysfunctional upbringings which can affect confidence may be:

- Brought up in a system outside of 'normal' e.g. religion, cult, education
- A parent with mental or physical health issues
- Somebody in the family with a health condition or disability
- Being of different ethnic origin to those in your community
- Moving home and school several times
- Parent with an addiction to alcohol, drugs or similar

- Brought up in poverty
- Not getting on well with a step-parent
- Parents arguing or fighting

Not all people who experience these challenges will lack confidence because we all deal with things differently. However, these situations may cause you to be in a very different situation to others around you. You become very aware of your differences. This can result in withdrawing from social interaction because it feels too awkward. You do not create friendships and feel isolated. This affects your self-belief and confidence.

Health issue or injury

Developing a health issue or an injury can seriously impact confidence. We are usually identified through what we do rather than who we are. I used to cycle race and was well known for this. This is how people identified with me although they only knew the competitive me, not the complete me. When I stopped racing, I felt as if part of my identity had disappeared.

If you are a keen sportsman and then develop a health issue or injury that stops you being able to do that activity, this can knock your confidence. During these times it can be useful to diversify. Rather than become deflated by what you cannot do, focus on what you can do. Since stopping cycling, I took up kart racing, am learning to play the keyboard and writing books. I see change as an opportunity, even if unplanned and not wanted.

Rather than looking at these challenges as the end of something, look upon them as the start of something new.

To develop as a person, it is important to take on new and different challenges. This way you learn more about yourself. There are many layers to each of us. Take the opportunity to uncover more layers as you broaden your knowledge or skills. You may surprise yourself.

When it comes to health or injury, I am not one to sit back and assume worst case scenario or believe that it has to stop me. I stopped cycling through undiagnosed chronic fatigue. I got to the point when I was feeling as if I would vomit every time I got on the bike. My body was telling me to stop on many levels. Recovery took me longer than I expected but now, I am so much better. I never gave up hope. I have not done things perfectly to regain my health but I am learning every step of the way.

When I have had injuries, I would read and research recovery methods. I recovered from golfer's elbow through supplementation and total commitment to recovery exercises. The same goes for knee and back injuries. My message to you is first and foremost, check out all options and believe you can recover. If someone tells you it takes 18 months to recover, do not take this as being the same for you. You might recover in a year or less. What you believe is important. The more positive and motivated you are, the more likely you will recover fully and quickly.

Work stress

Work stress can come in many forms. The most common reason for work-related stress is the quantity of work. Sometimes you believe that you should be able to cope with an enormous amount of work. Perhaps your boss suggests this to be the case. However, sometimes there are unrealistic expectations placed upon you.

In my experience, bosses will often leave the work to the people who say the least, keep their heads down and get on with it. They believe these people are coping just fine. The truth may be far from this. Therefore, it is your right and duty to advise your boss that the workload is too high and you need help. It is advisable to go in with a solution to the problem. Perhaps you create a plan to delegate or second someone over to help you out. Stand your ground and assert yourself because you have every right to make your boss aware of the problem.

Work stress may also be related to people. Bullying is one aspect covered already. Sometimes others annoy us or we have personality clashes. If this is unresolvable, moving department might be a solution. An alternative is to use Emotional Freedom Technique (Tapping) to clear your emotions about the challenging person or seek out help such as hypnotherapy.

Office politics and bureaucracy can create tremendous stress. This might be related to having too many chiefs or committees, colleagues being promoted undeservedly, unwanted changes in structure, meetings abouts meetings or dealing with colleagues who are useless at their job. Appraisal time can be an unwelcome stress too.

Perhaps you have to do presentations or talks. Public speaking anxiety is a problem for many people. Addressing this can make your work so much more enjoyable. The reason for this type of anxiety will most likely link in with past events, especially from childhood. It is also important to remember the reason you are asked to talk is because you know the subject and your audience wants to learn from you. Everyone listening is on your side and will want you to do well.

It is also absolutely fine not to know your entire subject. If asked a question you do not know the answer to, you can always say that you will get back to that person as you want to ensure you give them the correct information. It is also fine to say that, whatever the question, it is beyond your knowledge but that you will find out the answer or arrange for someone else to do so.

A big part of the fear of public speaking is the fear of appearing that you do not know the information but if you go in there with a plan for the questions you might not be able to answer, then you are prepared and will come across confident and in control. Thereby you will retain the attention of the audience. It is not always about what you do and do not know but how you respond when you do not have the answer.

Too much stress for long periods of time affects mental and physical health. Feeling you are not coping or others are doing better than you can impact confidence. It will most likely impact the quality of your sleep, which is vital to feeling good. Work is not worth taking your health away from you.

There may come a time when you need to consider moving jobs. You may not want to do this, especially if you are in a well-paid job, but consider the price you place on your well-being. Whatever the reason for staying in your job, bear in mind that your health is the most valuable asset you have. You can have more money than you need but if your health is suffering then your quality of life suffers too.

The problem with stressful jobs is the unhealthy ways people compensate and find ways to relax. This is sometimes done through drinking too much alcohol or other methods listed under the chapter on addiction. Work stress may lead to you not sleeping or eating well. You might stop exercising because you have little time available or feel exhausted. All of this frequently results in weight gain. High blood pressure can be a consequence of work pressures and an unhealthy lifestyle. If you find that you are reacting to work stress in an unhealthy manner or your confidence is impacted, then it is time to address it.

Redundancy/losing your job

Redundancy, being sacked or being forced out of a job can all cause a massive dent in your confidence. When you get the news, you will most likely be in shock, even if you had an insight it was coming. This would put you into the freeze response where consciousness shuts down. In that moment you are told you do not have a job, the information carries a strong emotional charge. Our physical body would absorb this information as a threat to our survival. This response also applies to other dramatic or shocking moments in our lives.

After the initial shock you may run through many scenarios in your mind. These may include:

- Needing to tell your partner/family.
- Will you get another job and if so, how soon?
- How could they do this to you?
- You've put so much of yourself into this job and this is how they repay you.
- How are you going to source sufficient funds to pay the mortgage/rent and get all the essentials?

- What will people think of you?

Along with this comes a mix of emotions from fear to anger. It is important, if you go through anything like this, that you form a plan of action to get back into work. This may involve updating your curriculum vitae (CV), re-training and applying for jobs. It may also be necessary to speak to your bank or landlord if funds are tight. If you have a partner, talk it all through with them. Go into problem-solving mode. You may need to make some financial adjustments. It is far better for your well-being to take action in these situations rather than fester and think about how bad the situation is.

Losing your job may be the best thing that happened to you. You might decide to take a sabbatical with the time between jobs and fulfil some ambitions or take time out for yourself to rebuild your energy or learn new skills.

It could be an opportunity to find employment in a field you enjoy, to work for a business that values you, to become self-employed or to have a less stressful job. Being forced into this position can be a blessing in disguise, as you can reassess your life and set new goals. In the moment something bad happens, it feels as if the world is closing in around you but out of every bad situation, an opportunity is just the other side.

In summary

There are many reasons why someone might lack confidence. The above gives you some insights to help you realise that life experiences go a long way to impacting how we feel about ourselves. Along with causing a lack of confidence, these issues can lead to anxiety or depression and other mental health challenges.

You can achieve far more than you realise by releasing those negative thoughts holding you back. Start to tell yourself you can do it. Later are some exercises which will help with confidence.

15. Finances

Financial pressures can be all-consuming. I have already mentioned how humans have evolved and that life was so much simpler only 40 years ago. Our financial needs were fairly basic back then. Priorities were to pay the mortgage or rent, utility bills, food, basic family car and school uniforms. If money was remaining, there could be an occasional treat such as an ice cream or fizzy drink. Birthday and Christmas presents were less extravagant back then. An annual family holiday was something the minority enjoyed.

Times have changed and with that has come more financial pressures than ever before. Nowadays people are spending over £1,000 on phones, buying expensive cars and clothes, mortgaging themselves to the hilt, holidays, hobbies, school fees, iPads, computers, gaming stations and more.

With technology forever changing, spending money can be an ever-demanding pressure. Add to this the temptation to run up store cards, credit cards and overdrafts, so many people do not have a clear understanding of their actual financial position.

If you are suffering financial pressures, you may need to consider changing your lifestyle. You will likely experience huge stress if your spending is out-weighing your income. If it is not creating stress, you are probably in denial and the stress will hit you at some point.

If you are living on the breadline, speak to people at Department for Work and Pensions or any other relevant department where you live. They will advise you if you are entitled to additional benefits. Also speak to a family member or trusted friend as they may help you out long enough to get back on your feet. It is important that you speak to someone and get some help. No-one would want you to be suffering.

I was brought up to spend only the money that is available. My parents were frugal and sensible with money and this seemed to rub off on to me. Here are a few simple tips which help to keep the stress levels down when it comes to finances:

- If you cannot afford it, do not buy it.

- When buying a property, record all your monthly expenses to ensure you can afford your mortgage. Also remember that most months there will be additional, unexpected, expenses so account for this.

- On the subject of mortgages. Sometimes people unnecessarily mortgage themselves to the hilt. This can create huge stress and sometimes cause you to be stuck in a job you loathe for years. We must remember that jobs are rarely for life nowadays. If you are in a highly paid job, give it plenty of thought before you dive in to a lot of debt.

- Do not spend because the money is there. You may not have a clue how long you will be on this earth for, but it takes the pressure off to know some spare funds are available for unexpected items.

- Consider annual costs. Most bills are Direct Debit and paid in monthly instalments but if you have an occasional yearly bill to pay, factor this in.

- If you are in the lower wage bracket, spend in alignment with your earnings. Expensive phones, for example, are an extravagance.

- Consider 'needs' over 'wants'.

- If you are self-employed, ensure you cover your social and tax expenses. I expect jurisdictions are different. In Guernsey, where I live, as a self-employed person, I pay my tax in two instalments on a six-monthly basis. If I fail to prepare for this, I might be in a financial mess. Therefore, each month I reserve what I need for my tax. Even though the money is still on my bank account until the time to pay it, as far as I am concerned it is in my income tax account and not for spending. I also put extra funds away in case I get an unexpected invoice. This happened to me a few years ago when I had a £2,000 social security bill.

- Keep on top of your finances. I still do old-fashioned bookkeeping on my accounts. I check my accounts weekly and keep a tally of spends. This way I am fully aware of my financial position. I am also aware if anything goes through my account which should not, such as a banking error or fraud.

- Save money whenever you can. It is a nice feeling seeing funds build up. There is the old saying "if you look after the pennies, the pounds will look after themselves". There is a lot of sense in this. I like certain luxuries and believe I work hard for them but understand that if times got tough, I could drop them. I balance this out with making some savings such as buying some items in bulk, buying some clothes in the sales and doing most of my own DIY.

- Do not ignore bills and invoices. Be efficient with them. In the same way I do a weekly account reconciliation to identify exactly where my finances stand, I also pay all my bills weekly. Some financial gurus may say leave your bills until the final day, but this leaves them niggling in the back of your head. Currently interest rates are so low and most current accounts are not paying anything so there is no gain to paying on the final demand.

- If you have loans in place at the moment, you may be able to consolidate them. Ensure you do this with a reputable institution and get a good interest rate.

- Shop around for insurance. Insurance companies can take your custom for granted but you can save yourself a lot of money by shopping around.

These are basic financial tips but have served me well in life.

I used to race bicycles for many years. Some racers would spend many thousands on new bikes every year. I never felt the need to do this. After all, bicycle technology does not change dramatically over the course of a year or two. I always saw my bike as a tool to do a job.

The same with phones. One of my tech-minded friends was belittling my phone because it was out of date in his view. As I told him, I really did not care because it did everything I needed it to do.

There is often competitiveness amongst men when it comes to materialistic items such as cars, phones and other 'toys'.

It is as if the materialistic items define them or their status in life. In fact, I do recall one male client saying to me that his car was an indication of his level of success. This philosophy sometimes causes men to get into debt in order to keep up with their friends or colleagues. Women do this too; just in case you were about to lynch me!

The last finance job I had was run by two very down-to-earth people. One of whom still had the same car he had purchased 15 years earlier. It did not matter to him what car he drove, even though he was partial owner of a successful financial business and could afford something much more deluxe.

Striving to keep up with others on materialistic items is a cumbersome task. People who like to show off their value through materialistic items are trying to make a statement of the type of person they are. All the materialistic stuff is shop window dressing. It does not reflect the person you are. Your actions and what you say reflect the kind of person you are. If buying the latest, greatest and best is something you feel obligated to do, set yourself free now.

Surely happiness is the best way to define success? Spending money on materialistic items brings short term happiness, whereas there are many ways to find true joy in life which are priceless. For me, this would include spending time with my cats, listening to music, having a laugh with friends or walking in nature. All of these have a deeper sensation of self-nurture and work wonders with the body to de-stress.

Most pleasures in life come from the simple things such as walking along the beach, riding your bike through the countryside, taking your dog for a walk, coffee with a friend, binge-watching a television series or reading a book.

With all of this said, if one of your real pleasures in life is having a new car or £10,000 bicycle, by all means go for it. However, please do not think you must do so in order to keep up with others. Do it for you and only if you have the funds available.

Importantly do not spend to impress anyone. It is your business what you spend your money on and how you control your finances. Owing money is stressful and when it goes as far as being summonsed to court the problem becomes very real.

It is a good feeling to save money and to see the figures going higher in your bank account. This gives you comfort and peace of mind too. Even if you are a high earner, you should be conscious of your spending to ensure you are making sound financial decisions and fully aware of your financial position. Many high earners end up in financial ruin as institutions happily loan them huge amounts of money, which they fail to repay.

In summary, understand your financial position and never ignore debt because it only increases if not attended to. Check your bank accounts at least weekly and be prepared for any payments that will go through them, especially annual payments, Direct Debits and such like.

If finance is not your thing, I encourage you to seek help so you can learn how to take charge of your own budget better. If you have a trustworthy friend or family member who is good with finances, ask them for some guidance. It can save you many headaches to know where your financial position is at any time.

16. Self-acceptance

It is common for anybody with mental health issues to feel bad about themselves. Likewise, having such negative opinions of yourself creates poor mental health. This becomes a vicious cycle of negativity. Most people who have depression have negative thoughts and experience self-doubt. Men often believe they should be strong and pull themselves together.

You also assume that you are weak or strange because you think other men are not going through the same challenges you are. This causes additional, and often severe, internal rumblings of negativity within yourself. In reality, at some point in their life, most men will experience a mental health challenge even if they do not identify it as such. This is because of the life we lead in this modern world and the pressures of day-to-day life.

You are in a vast and varied club with many brilliant people. You could say you are in the majority rather than a minority. Not as you thought, right? You assumed you were the odd one out, the weird one, the useless and incapable one. Well, that's just not the case. It is important that you understand and accept this.

Just like you, other men are very good at hiding their mental health issues and many hate to admit they are experiencing them or have done in the past. However, hundreds of thousands of men are experiencing a mental health challenge right now. Sometimes these are manageable, and other times they are overwhelming.

Lack of self-acceptance is a powerful feature of such

issues. The negative thoughts you have towards yourself are incorrect. They do not reflect fairly the wonderful and capable person you are. The issue exacerbates because it becomes difficult to get those negative thoughts out of your head and you reconfirm them every time you repeat them.

The thought processing goes something like this:

*It is difficult to accept yourself when you cannot **control** the way you feel. After all, a man should be in **control**.*

*You feel **powerless** to this behaviour and these thoughts, which results in a negative opinion of yourself. After all, a man should feel **powerful**.*

*Self-acceptance is impossible because the way you are feeling suggests you are **weak**. After all, a man is meant to be **strong**.*

And so on.....

This thought process creates huge internal conflict for you. Your view on self-acceptance comes down to what you believe should be the standard behaviour for men and the archetypal man. Based on my explanation of the evolution of man, we can see a mismatch between these deep core beliefs, which are part of your DNA, and the reality of the society we live in.

We need to set a new baseline which allows you to speak about the stresses of life, feel your emotions and be your unique and wonderful self with no need to conform to any archetype of man.

There may be other reasons for your lack of self-acceptance. As with many of our bad feelings towards ourselves, this can be an issue rooted back to our past. If you were told negative things about yourself, you may well have believed them, especially if you were told them over and over. If you thought you were a failure, ugly, stupid or held other unhelpful opinions of yourself then those would cause you to have a low level of self-acceptance.

You may berate yourself for some of your past behaviour. You cannot physically go back into the past to change those events, but you can recognise that you are an ever-changing person. If we are honest, at least 90% of us are not proud of things we have done in the past, but living with regret will never change that past behaviour.

I could list you a number of things I am not proud of or would do differently now given another opportunity. However, I accept that most of these situations were during my youth, when I may not have considered the consequences of my actions or have the knowledge and resources to deal with events in the way I do now.

Sometimes I may have acted out of a moment of spontaneity or through rebellion. Despite these actions, I know I am not a bad person. I know this because I care for people and animals; I do good things and have a good heart. The past is just that. It does not dictate who you are now. The action you take now and in the future are better indications of the person you are.

Even if you did do a terrible act, you can now do positive acts of kindness or decide how you grow as a person. We are here to develop. I put my effort into improving myself as a person. This means, either improving in a way that enables me to help others or creating a better life to bring me more peace and happiness.

If you have behaved in a way that you now regret, the best thing you can do for yourself is to gain some understanding of that behaviour. Perhaps at the time you lacked self-respect, direction or support. It is also important to acknowledge that you are not that same person you were back then. This applies even if this event happened a week or a month ago.

We continue to change, learn and develop. We change through the information we absorb and how we process and use such information. We are here on earth to learn and grow through wisdom and to create a better life for our human race. Use those past situations as a platform to make your world or someone else's world a better place in any way you can that is congruent with the person you are.

If you need to apologise to make things right, then do it. A heartfelt apology, even if 20 years late, is a worthwhile apology; whether or not it is accepted. You cannot be responsible for whether the person on the receiving end accepts the apology. Therefore, relinquish any need for acceptance. The important point is to make the apology but only if heartfelt.

When we focus outward by helping others, we put our energy to good use and create a positive focus. This can help with your mental health. This is why ex-drug addicts will speak in schools to discourage children from doing the same. It serves as part of their healing process and helps to build their own self-acceptance and respect.

One challenge of depression is not having the energy or motivation to take action. With anxiety you fear taking action. Take small steps to start with when you feel ready. Giving back is valuable but doing so in a way that does not drain your energy or take too much from you is important. Keep a good level of balance. Do not ignore self-preservation when aiming to help others.

17. Medication

Whether or not to take medication for mental health issues can be a challenging consideration. As I am not a physician, I cannot tell you what to do with regard to medication. I will tell you what I have learned from my clients.

There are times, perhaps for a period of time or occasionally for life, when medication is needed to create sufficient stability to enable you to address the underlying issues and to function in life.

Nowadays there is a growing awareness that taking synthetic medication is not always good. Many people do not wish to be taking it long term, if at all. When you receive your packet of medication, it will tell you about possible side effects. If you are a hypochondriac, reading the list could cause you to worry. Bear in mind though, that you might not experience any of the side effects mentioned on the list.

Medication is not a solution or fix for mental health issues. At best it relieves the symptoms and allows people to function normally. I should mention, that if you do decide to come off medication, please do so under the guidance of your physician. If you suddenly stop taking medication it can cause very unpleasant detoxification effects as your mind and body adjust.

As a consequence of taking medication for mental health issues, such as depression and anxiety, clients have reported a range of symptoms to me, including feeling emotionally numb, therefore unable to experience positive emotions, gastrointestinal issues, nausea and dizziness. Occasionally more unusual symptoms have been reported to me.

In many cases, medication is not required. Addressing the underlying issues, which are causing the mental health issues, can provide that much-needed resolution. You do not need to know or understand those underlying issues right now. The therapist you work with is set with the task of uncovering and addressing the root causes.

You may wonder whether you can recover without any outside assistance. That depends on you. I always urge people who experience severe trauma or abuse to work with a professional. If anything feels too challenging or causes you to feel huge fear or overwhelmed at the thought of addressing it, I encourage you to seek professional help.

When a patient seeks help from their GP for mental health issues, it seems that medication is often handed out rather swiftly. The questions I would love people to be asked are:

"What is going on in your life, which is causing you stress or upset?"
"What has changed in your life recently?"
"What was happening for you around the time the symptoms began?"

In summary, there is no definitive answer to whether you take medication. It depends completely on your own personal situation. This is for you to discuss with your physician if you wish. It may also depend on other options available to you.

18. Childhood abuse

Childhood abuse occurs in different forms including neglect, sexual abuse, physical and emotional abuse. As a society we often focus more on the abuse of girls and women. This may result in boys and men thinking the abuse they suffer is less significant or important. You may also believe you should have done something at the time to stop it. This adds to all the negative feelings and beliefs you hold about yourself.

If you have suffered any abuse as a child, there is no doubt, it will significantly impact your life and the person you are.

Anyone who has been abused will usually hold a low opinion of themselves, feel insecure and have a huge amount of self-doubt. It can cause you to struggle throughout life in terms of school, relationships and careers. Of course, you may be successful in many areas of life, such as sport or career, but often that success is driven by unresolved trauma and blocked emotions. That drive can come from an unhealthy place and cause irrational behaviour.

Men who have suffered abuse will rarely talk about it through shame, guilt or embarrassment.

Abuse can come from many different people: a parent, sibling, step-mother or father, teacher, sports coach, social club leader, friends, other family members, church or many other situations. As children, we are vulnerable, very trusting and an easy target for abusers.

Sexual abuse leaves overwhelming mental scars. There are so many tough aspects to this. Often you keep the abuse a secret. This may be for different reasons:

- You did not expect to be believed if you spoke up, so you kept quiet about it.
- You were confused about the situation at the time and thought what happened was okay because you were told this to be the case.
- You were told you led the perpetrator on. Therefore, it was your fault.
- You may not want to hurt your parents by telling them, so you carry the burden alone.
- You were told by the perpetrator that it is 'your little secret' to be kept between you.
- The perpetrator told you that if you tell anyone you will go to prison or they will hurt you or your family.
- You think it was all your fault, you are to blame and carry a feeling of disgust towards yourself for life.
- You may not know who to tell as you have lost all trust.
- You may be in fear of telling anyone because you do not know what will happen.
- If a close family member abused you, you may be worried about speaking up because you do not want them to go to prison.
- As a child you feared being removed from your family.
- You were told that you enjoyed it which caused you to believe you were responsible.

As well as low self-esteem, abuse in any form can cause anxiety and depression. It can lead to addictive behaviour, anger issues, OCD, self-harm, and any of the other issues mentioned in this book. Personality disorders are sometimes diagnosed following abuse.

Abuse in any form is destructive. If you have come through abuse then you are a hero. If you are struggling with life after abuse, I urge you to seek help. Abuse is not something you can deal with on your own.

If you were abused, it was not your fault. I have known people, now adults, continue to hold themselves responsible for the abuse they suffered as a young child. Knowing abuse is wrong, without any doubt whatsoever, as an adult does not stop you holding negative beliefs about yourself which were formed years ago.

When I ask someone, who has been abused this question, it changes how they see the situation: "how can that 7-year-old child be held responsible?" When you think of a 7-year-old child (or whatever age is relevant), and separate yourself from the child, you realise how vulnerable and naive they were. No child can be held responsible for the abuse they suffer. Never!

Another aspect of this issue is witnessing abuse. I have known youngsters witness their mother being hit by their father or step-father. As a young child there is nothing they can do, although they want to protect their mother. This can go on for years and ruin their childhood. It can leave you feeling helpless and useless and believing you are pathetic for not doing something. However, reality is that a young boy could never stand up to a grown man and come off on top.

Witnessing abuse can be as damaging as experiencing it because you most likely freeze through the trauma and form negative beliefs about yourself in that moment. Guilt can be a common feeling for those in this situation. Guilt that you did not act, guilt that you hid out of sight of the abuser, guilt that you did not get hurt when others did or guilt for not speaking up. There is one person who should feel guilty and that is the person carrying out the attack. No child should ever have to witness such acts. Once again, if this or similar has happened to you then you need a massive pat on the back for making it this far.

Emotional abuse can involve being told you are useless, leaving you feeling you are incapable. This will ruin your self-esteem and confidence. It might involve threatening behaviour which could potentially materialise into physical harm. The threat in itself is abuse.

There are many forms of emotional abuse. As a child you may have experienced some of the following:

- Being told you are ugly, fat or any other derogatory term.
- Derogatory pet names e.g.: "my chubby bear"
- You can never do anything right e.g. "you messed up again", "you're useless".
- Embarrass you in public, e.g. telling others personal things about you or belittling you.
- Intimidating behaviour such as shouting in your face, hovering over you or swearing at you.
- Putting you down or making fun of anything you do or achieve.
- Threatening you by telling you things they will do to you.
- Threatening to send you to a children's home away from your entire family.

Physical abuse as a child also comes in different forms. I have noted some examples below:

- Biting
- Hitting, either with hands or objects
- Punching
- Holding down in a position from which you cannot move

Stresses of Modern Man

- Starving
- Overly forceful handling
- Hair pulling
- Kicking
- Scratching
- Shaking
- Slapping
- Throwing the child
- Burning or scalding
- Anything torturous such as pushing head under water or being made to stand in a cold and dark shed for hours with no food, water or toilet facilities.
- Neglect is also physically abusive.

Some parents may abuse a child physically because they were brought up in a similar manner and see it as normal behaviour. Others may do so because they cannot control their anger. Some people abuse to incite fear.

Childhood neglect leaves long term emotional scars. It can also cause lifelong physical health issues. One key area which may not be seen as significant is the emotional neglect. It is important that children feel listened to and their emotions and feelings are validated. For example, if they were upset by a friend's actions, a parent should listen to their thoughts and acknowledge them. They may put forth a new perspective to help the child bring new understanding to the situation. It is important, though, to acknowledge the child's grievance on the matter.

Sometimes the parents have their own problems, including mental health issues, substance abuse, addictions, physical health problems or may have suffered neglect as a child themselves.

If a child's emotional needs are neglected, they will grow up with a lack of self-worth, self-esteem and confidence. They will be unlikely to speak up and prefer to hide themselves away. There may be giveaway signs of this which can be noticed by teachers or other adults in their social environment. The child may become withdrawn or anxious, skip school, give up trying either in terms of school work or in hobbies or start to behave badly. This can escalate into more severe issues such as self-harming or substance abuse.

Neglect involves the following:

- Failing to respond to a child's emotional needs.
- Failure to provide food or water.
- Lack of education.
- Lack of interest in the child and their life.
- Failure to ensure the child is clean and has clean clothes.
- Exposing the child to unsuitable scenes either on television, internet or in person, e.g. alcohol or drug abuse, sexual or physical violence. This would also be emotional and, in some cases, sexual abuse.
- Failure to provide suitable clothing and shoes.
- Lack of involvement in the child's life.
- Leaving the child alone or without appropriate supervision.
- Unsuitable sleeping environment.
- A dirty or unsafe home environment.
- Failure to provide or seek adequate health care (including dental care)

Many people who have suffered abuse hold a low opinion of themselves. They will often hold themselves to blame because they may well have been told they did wrong. The beliefs we form as children, do not just disappear when we become adults. This is despite having the knowledge and freedom to know better as adults. However, those beliefs can be addressed so you start to feel so much better. You can release the negative emotions you have held for years and begin the process of building up your confidence and self-esteem.

Every child born into this world has a right to a loving home and to live free from fear. Abuse in any form will leave you with deeply held trauma, both in your subconscious mind and the cells of your body. Through certain therapies, this trauma can be healed.

If you suffered any childhood abuse, it is important to appreciate the amazing person you are. You are still here, trying to make a better life for yourself. To make it this far proves you are an incredible resourceful and resilient person. You may not feel or believe this is the case but I assure you it is.

It is important to acknowledge that you were a child when the abuse happened. What on earth can a child do? That child did not fully understand the situation. They could not fully understand the right and the wrong. They may have been told it is a secret, it is normal or they would get hurt or lose their family if they spoke about it. As children we do not have a full perspective on the rights and wrongs of life. We absorb the information we are told. We are vulnerable and trust adults to take care of us. The child is never responsible for any abuse they may have endured, never.

The short-term and long-term effects of child abuse include:

- Feeling powerless
- Believe the abuse is their fault

- Confused
- Bed-wetting
- Self-judgement
- Distrust
- Behavioural issues
- Anger and violence
- Lack of self-esteem and confidence
- Failed relationships
- Mental health issues
- Develop unhealthy coping mechanisms
- Self-sabotage
- Physical health issues

People who experience abuse of any form as a child are more likely to go into abusive relationships. This is due to their lack of self-esteem, self-worth and confidence. They are often vulnerable as adults, continuing to be a victim. Sometimes the victim becomes the perpetrator.

Exercise - write a letter to younger self

When we get older and have the benefit of life experiences, we may wish we had understood ourselves and the experiences we had as a child differently. We may have liked to have told our younger self that they were clever and capable. We want them to know they were a good boy. Perhaps they needed to know that they would be loved later in life.

It can be an incredibly healing exercise to write a letter to your younger self telling them all the things you wish you had known and understood back then.

Whether or not you were abused, give this a go now. You can add to it later on if you wish. Tell them what they will achieve, that they are a good person and that they are loved. Tell that child everything you wish you had known when you were younger. To help you, I have prepared an example letter in the Appendix.

19. Relationship issues

Decades ago, people would get married and stay together until one of the them departed the earth. This does not mean they were happy in their relationship. In many cases, quite the contrary. Affairs happened, arguments occurred, abuse too and people struggled with their sexuality or gender. People experienced mental health issues but it was all hushed up and a facade portrayed to the world.

In more recent times, if people are unhappy in a relationship, they are less likely to stay together. They move on and form new relationships. This has led to more complicated family structures and dealing with issues of affairs, divorces, split families, arguments with ex's, custody battles, financial worries, countless emotions, regrets and so on. All of this can take its toll.

I could fill an entire book on the subject of relationships. However, we have so much to cover on other topics. Therefore, for now, I offer you some insights and fresh perspectives.

Relationship break-up

If you go through a relationship split, the best advice I can give you is to aim for an amicable separation, especially if it involves children. It is rare to come out of a relationship in a majestic place. For most people, there is a period of healing to undergo.

Relationship break-up involving children

The most important thing is to give your children the best life and to show them you both can get on, with the children's interests at the core of any settlements and arrangements.

With a little give and take on each side, life is easier all round. There will be frustrations. Ignore the minor things that niggle you about your ex-partner's parenting and only address those issues which concern you because, in some way, it is not good for your child. When you address it, you are more likely to get your ex-partner on side if you do so in the most positive way.

I suggest you start the conversation with a positive and include the reason why you feel the way you do so it shows you have your child's best interests at heart. This can lead to a more amicable way forward in co-parenting. For example, "Julie enjoyed her day at the beach with you on Sunday. I am wondering if you would bring her home by 5 pm in future, so that she has time for tea and can get ready for school the next day? She was rather exhausted on Monday and was nearly late for school."

In the above example, there is the positive "Julie enjoyed her day at the beach with you on Sunday", followed by the request which is specific "I am wondering if you would bring her home by 5 pm in future so that she has time for tea and get ready for school the next day?" and the reason behind it "she was rather exhausted on Monday and was nearly late for school." The tone in which you speak is important too. Therefore, keep to a positive and light tone - even if you are seething.

I am not who I was

Put simply - we change. If I look back at myself through every decade of my life, I have changed. Sometimes when we are in a relationship, we both grow but in completely opposite directions. We grow to a level that does not enable that relationship to continue harmoniously. There is no right or wrong in this. There is no need to point a finger in your direction or in anyone else's. Change is what we do. How boring life would be if we never learned from any experience, never did new things and continued to live life without getting to know ourselves better?

We change partly through life experiences. I look at what I do now in terms of how I live my life, the career I have and the people I connect with. I could never have expected any of this when I was 20 years old. I am far more introverted than I was then or perhaps I am now honouring the introvert in me.

Change is not wrong either. Sometimes, with change comes pain, especially if it means that a relationship is not working. Sometimes one partner will say, "it's not you it's me." This is because they recognise that their needs and wants have changed in a way that no longer fits the relationship. Honour the changes you make in life. As you change and explore yourself and life more, you are becoming a more complete version of yourself.

Affairs

Affairs will always create huge upset. At the time an affair starts, there is no intention to create that upset or hurt anyone but inevitably it will happen. If you have been affected by an affair, whichever end you were on, the receiving end or the perpetrator, then this will most likely impact your well-being due to the stress involved. How much of an impact depends on so many factors.

If you hold on to negative emotions, I encourage you to work through these. Sometimes couples can work through their difficulties and stay together following an affair but very often the relationship is never the same as it was previously. Affairs can come between people decades after they happened even if they stay together.

Trust can be an issue. If you were on the receiving end, you may find it difficult to trust any future partner but this can be worked through. Live in the moment. None of us know what the future holds, so surely it is best to enjoy the present? Living in fear that a new partner will do the same will stop you enjoying the new relationship fully and cause tension between you and your partner. Decide to enjoy each day for what it brings. Your relationship has a better chance of blossoming if you do this.

Wasted years

People often talk in terms of regrets when it comes to ending relationships. They believe the years they were together are meaningless and therefore have wasted those years. This is not the case. You did not waste those years, you lived them.

At the end of a relationship is a lot of emotional pain. You will run through many situations in your mind. You will recall past events and wonder what the future holds. Over time the pain will lessen. You may even realise that, to finish the relationship, was for the best.

Life is full of many experiences as if chapters of a book. Each chapter is full and varied. If a relationship ended, it was the end of that particular chapter for you and there is always a blank page ready to start something bright and new, with you as the author.

You have an opportunity to learn from past relationships. Where do you believe they went wrong? What has changed about you in those years? How do you want your life to be in the future?

You could say that finishing a relationship enables you to enter a new relationship, which can be more joyful and fulfilling.

In many cases, time does seem to be a healer. Creating new, more fulfilling relationships is the light at the end of a dark tunnel. Likewise, you may be perfectly content on your own.

Partner and career

If your partner has a career which means they earn more money than you or they are considered more successful, this may cause you to have feelings of low self-esteem or lack of confidence and self-worth. It may cause you to feel insecure or worthless.

Any idea that men are the main breadwinners in a family are outdated. Some women can be incredibly determined to fulfil their chosen career path. Sometimes when one partner is so driven, the other person in the relationship makes sacrifices to their own career. It is important to consider that relationships are partnerships, each person playing their role to make the partnership and family unit work at its best. A career is just one aspect of that.

Each of you serves a unique role in your relationship. You may be the one who gives your time more freely or is more flexible.

You may do more DIY or cook. You may be the one to create laughter or who does more with the children. These are all aspects of a relationship. Each of you need to contribute. This contribution will relate to many different aspects of the relationship. It is not all about the career you have or the amount of money you earn. Happiness is priority. Without happiness in a relationship something needs to change.

There may also be times when it appears that one of you is supporting the other more. Not just in financial terms but perhaps emotional support. Relationships are not about the scales being balanced completely. A good relationship is when the scales might tilt one way and then the other. It is about pulling through together without pointing the finger or looking for payback.

Family trauma

Sometimes in life we, or a member of our family, go through something traumatic. This might be something that rocks the entire family. It can pull a family closer together or tragically tear them apart. People deal with trauma in different ways. Some will throw themselves into their job, charity work or some other cause. A number may drink themselves to oblivion and others may bottle everything up and have a massive breakdown 10 years later.

This is a huge topic, too big for this book, but my advice to you is to address trauma through a professional and encourage family members to do the same. Trauma rarely goes away without finding its way back to the surface. There is never a convenient time to address these issues so do not wait for the right time. Now is a good time.

Respect, happiness, partnership

There are many elements to a good relationship. At the core of relationships should be respect, happiness and working as a partnership. Sometimes when relationships start to go sour there is a pulling apart. One or both of you react to behaviour of your partner which irritates you. You begin to lose patience and shout at each other.

I remember a friend telling me that her and her ex-partner "knew how to push each other's buttons". I commented "why would you do that?". This made no sense to me. If we want to be with someone, surely we want a harmonious relationship rather than deliberately creating angst, frustration and arguments.

Let us look at these three words in turn:

Respect

In terms of relationships, respect is a two-way thing. Here are some examples of when respect is not shown:

- Your partner being derogatory towards you
- Not doing their fair share of chores (this depends on other factors such as work, etc but 'fair' is the key word here based on what you have agreed)
- Disregarding your feelings
- Putting themselves first
- Not treating you as an equal
- Not allowing you to have your own opinion
- Controlling behaviour
- Not allowing you freedom/time to yourself or to be with friends
- Believing they own you

- Not supporting each other
- Mental abuse
- Undermining confidence
- Physical abuse

Some of the above will also fall into the 'abuse' category.

Respect works both ways. If someone is trying to control you or does not trust you, most likely they have underlying issues. Some people go from one abusive relationship to another abusive relationship. This is often because they lack self-esteem, self-worth or self-confidence. Abuse often starts slowly with small negative gestures. Stopping unacceptable behaviour immediately is important. Make it absolutely clear that is it not acceptable, otherwise the issue escalates and has potential to become serious.

Happiness

What is a relationship without happiness? Sometimes we get so used to having the other person in our lives, going to work and leading a busy life that we forget to laugh together or appreciate the other person. This is harder when you have families because pressures are higher and time is more limited.

This is why some relationships do not continue until death do us part. One or both partners realises the happiness has gone. Either as a partner or a family, ensure you share some quality happy time. The best way to achieve this is to do things together. Sometimes this can be a simple event, such as watching a movie, having a takeaway, playing a game or going for a walk. Consider what makes you and your partner happy and ensure you create some joy together in life.

Partnership

Working together in partnership to help and support each other is critical. I have found relationships to work well when playing to each other's strengths rather than criticising where we fall short. Also doing some chores together can be good because it gives you the feeling of teamwork. For example:

- Cooking
- Gardening
- DIY
- Cleaning vehicles

I'm sure you can get the idea from the above. Also split other chores to play to your strengths. For example, I do all the financials and paperwork side of things because my husband will leave paperwork, which stresses me out. Therefore, I remove the stress by doing this side of things. However, on the flip side of this, he does a lot of the out of house chores such as the shopping. I am most happy at home but he likes to get out and about.

It is far better to divide chores based on each of your strengths rather than get frustrated when your partner does not do certain things or do them how you want them completed. Divide and conquer the chores in your relationship together. With this, we bear in mind 'respect'.

Partnership also involves doing some pleasant things together. I have always found relationships better when my partner and I do an activity together. Sometimes this has been as simple as going for a walk and other times it might be cycling or a swim at the beach.

On the contrary, living in each other's pockets, so you have no personal time to yourself, is not necessarily healthy for a relationship either. This is because we should recognise our individual needs and freedom. However, doing some activities together keeps the relationship alive.

Partnership is also about talking and listening. For some people, this is challenging. This might be because as a youngster, you could not express your emotions, thoughts or feelings. However, being able to talk about your concerns, worries, problems or anything else with your partner keeps everything honest and it means they understand you and what you are going through.

If you keep all your thoughts and worries inside, this can leave your partner wondering what you are thinking. They might start to assume all kinds of things are going on. Of course, their assumptions could be completely wrong. This is why honest communication is always best. I would much rather know if my husband was worried or annoyed about something. That way I understand if he is a little withdrawn or loses his temper easily. I can also provide a listening ear and some support or perhaps some advice or new perspectives. There is much to be gained on both sides from communicating.

If you hide away the fact that you are struggling and one day lose your temper completely or have a breakdown, your partner may not have seen it coming. Even if you do not understand what you are feeling or why you are feeling that way tell them that something is not right.

Our past

As with everything else in life, our relationships are affected by our past. The same goes for you and your partner. Therefore, if either of you are struggling, consider whether it is related to a situation happening currently in your life or could it be to do with something from your past causing you to react in an unhealthy way. If it is not the former, it is likely to be the latter, i.e. the past. If this is the case then be prepared to get the issue addressed. That way you will feel so much better for it and it will enhance your relationship.

In summary

It is impossible to address every relationship issue in this book but the above should give you some guidance. It is too easy to get stuck in a rut of unhappiness. Nevertheless, we should be happy most of the time. We do not need to be jumping with joy or walking around with a silly grin on our faces but we should be feeling safe, content and have a good laugh sometimes.

Communication helps a relationship along. Never assume your partner knows what is going on in your head. Providing support for each other in all kinds of situations can be hugely beneficial. Take time out for you both to ensure that quality time becomes a part of life.

20. ADHD and ASD

Attention-deficit hyperactivity disorder (ADHD) and autism spectrum disorder (ASD) can present a variety of challenges. The most common of those are related to friendship groups, relationships, socialising and the workplace. The severity of these disorders can be dramatically different from person to person.

To achieve a diagnosis for ADHD requires a detailed evaluation. Most children are not diagnosed until school age. Many people never obtain a diagnosis, whilst others are diagnosed later in life. For many a diagnosis gives them some comfort because they can make sense of their behaviour and the challenges it presents.

Many men with these issues will also suffer with anxiety. They may have experienced bullying. Their place of work might not be empathetic to the challenges faced by someone with ASD or ADHD. Therefore, can be unwilling to make adjustments.

Let's look at these in a little more detail.

ADHD is defined by an ongoing pattern of inattention and/or hyperactivity-impulsivity that interferes with functioning or development.

Common traits of ADHD are:

- Easily distracted from the task at hand.
- Make careless mistakes.
- Struggle to follow instructions.
- Difficulty in sequencing tasks.
- Short attention span.

- Forgetful.
- Struggle to maintain focus and see a project through.
- Disorganised.
- Appear fidgety.
- Takes hasty action (without considered thought).
- Socially intrusive.
- Low social awareness.
- More likely to say what they think rather than speak with consideration for others.
- Lose things.
- Be overly talkative.
- Not monitor their volume of speech.
- Too quick to respond if they know the answer (not let the other person finish).
- Appear overly energetic.

ASD is a developmental disorder which influences communication and behaviour. Nowadays it can be diagnosed in the first two years of life, although for some is still diagnosed later. Diagnosis is achieved through an assessment process.

Common traits of ASD are:

- Difficulty with communication and interaction with other people.
- Restricted interests.
- Make little or inconsistent eye contact.
- May not pay attention to others.
- Struggle to connect with others and form relationships.
- Fail to, or be slow to, respond to someone calling their name or to other verbal attempts to gain attention.
- Struggle with conversation.
- May go into great detail on a subject they are passionate

about.
- Contradictory facial expressions and gestures to what they are saying or thinking.
- Tone of voice may be unusual.
- May create repetitive behaviours.
- Can become absorbed in passions and retain data in great detail.
- Struggle to deal with changes in routine. This may cause them to become anxious or emotional. Although for some, routine can be challenging.
- Can be overwhelmed with sensory input from any of the senses.

I have worked with several men diagnosed with high-functioning autism; this is the term used to refer to those on the autistic spectrum but have good intellectual abilities and can generally function day to day very well. They are very capable, although may struggle with emotional intelligence, relationships and experience social challenges.

Asperger's Syndrome (Asperger's) was incorporated under the ASD umbrella in 2013 in the Diagnostic and Statistical Manual of Mental Disorders 5th Edition (DSM-5). Therefore, all diagnoses, whether pre or post the 2013 consolidation, come under the umbrella "autism spectrum disorder". However, some people still use the term Asperger's Syndrome and identify more easily with this term. For this reason, I have identified this separately here.

Men with Asperger's can function very well in many areas of life. However, social situations and relationships can be very challenging. It creates communication challenges and lack of emotional awareness or understanding.

Someone with Asperger's can come across as harsh, as if they have no interest in your feelings or desires. They can also become good actors, mimicking behaviour they know a new partner would expect but over time this behaviour fades because it is hard work maintaining the pretence. At this point, the relationship becomes strained.

Many traits of Asperger's will be familiar from the ASD list of traits. Most notably, someone with Asperger's would show the following characteristics:

- A lack of social and emotional awareness.
- Find social situations challenging, even torturous.
- Long-term friendships or relationships are difficult to form.
- Will have black and white thinking.
- Can unwittingly cause upset due to lack of emotional consideration and understanding when in discussion.
- Typically copes well with structure and routine. Although some find routine tedious.
- Not comfortable with spontaneity. This can cause, what appears to be, an irrational response from someone with Asperger's.
- Can shut down midway through a conversation.
- Have obsessive interests and talk in great detail about them. This is irrelevant of whether the person they are talking to is interested or completely bored.
- Appear to lack empathy. Often because they do not express empathy as others do.
- Tend to like statistics, figures and facts rather than discussions around thoughts and feelings.
- Small talk is mind-blowingly boring. They are likely to show their disinterest.
- Can come across as too honest or harsh due to a lack of emotional filter.

- Enjoy time alone and may need this in order to re-energise.

In the right career, the challenges of Asperger's are not a problem. People with Asperger's will usually move towards a suitable career path. In today's age, there are more career opportunities for people expressing traits of Asperger's than ever before with computer technicians, web designers, application developers, engineers and scientists being excellent career paths and in high demand.

People with Asperger's often have incredible focus and can be determined and persistent. They can be very good at seeing a task through to the end and are great solution providers in the right environment. They often pick out detail that others will not notice. In fact, excellent attention to detail is an Asperger's trait.

Close relationships can be more demanding though. Although, in the right partnership, someone with Asperger's can have a great relationship. This requires understanding and acceptance of your behaviours from your partner.

A diagnosis can help you both gain greater insight into ASD. Having said all this, if you are both happy and understand that the traits are not a deliberate way of being difficult or not caring then you may not feel a diagnosis will serve you any purpose. It is your call.

People with ADHD or ASD may have different challenges but will often suffer anxiety and are at risk of depression. This is because they find the social side of life challenging or they find it difficult to fit into structures such as the workplace or clubs. This can cause them to feel isolated.

Stress can be a trigger for ASD behaviour, making it more intense. Bullying can be common, which can dent confidence and self-esteem. This can cause them to want to stay in the safe environment of home. They may feel lonely and have few, if any, friends.

If ever anyone is judging you for having one of these conditions, please understand that they are ignorant. I mean that in the nicest possible way. They may have no idea you have the condition. Of course, this is still no reason to judge but they might be kinder if they knew your behaviour was due to one of these challenges. Some people will judge anyway. This says more about them than it does about you. Do not let their attitude become your problem.

I have found when working with clients with these challenges, it is important to find methods that work specifically for them. A real positive is they are very good at telling me when something is not working for them so then we move on. They often benefit from some simple relaxation techniques, such as deep breathing, but also from positive affirmations.

It is important for them to know they can come into a safe and non-judgmental environment and talk about anything on their mind. Through my work, I have seen a number of teenage boys with ADHD or ASD. They talk about their relationship struggles and how they find it difficult to make friends or form loving relationships.

If you have any of these conditions, it should not stop you achieving your aims and goals in life. It is also possible to have a lovely personal relationship and good friends. There can be positives to these conditions because the mind works in different ways. This means you can develop a strong skill set utilising your natural abilities. As long as you are passionate about something and follow it through, then you have a great opportunity to be successful.

It is advisable to make people aware you have the condition because they can then have some understanding. Explain your challenges to your workplace, friends and family. If we make people more aware then we are spreading knowledge and creating awareness of very common conditions.

Having these conditions makes you no less capable than anyone else. People with ADHD or ASD are very likeable too. In reality, we can all float across the spectrum. When we are stressed, we may show stronger traits than when we are relaxed and content.

Along with other holistic help such as hypnotherapy and tapping, Rhythmic Movement Training (RMT) is a treatment which can help with the challenges of ADHD and ASD. RMT was developed as a movement-based treatment to integrate retained reflexes. More details on RMT are contained under the section on therapy options.

Below are comments I received from a reader who was diagnosed later in life with autism:

"You are totally spot on when you talk about people with ASD struggling socially, in the work place, with friendship groups and relationships. I have made friends easily and sincerely, only for many of these friendships to evaporate. This leaves me puzzled and confused, then depressed and anxious about making new friends. I guess my behaviour, at times, did not comply with accepted norms, unstated stuff.

When I ask for explanations, I am told that everything is fine, and that nothing has changed, yet I no longer see the friends in question. That said, I am blessed in having friends who have stuck with me through it all. Recently, following my assessment, I went to tell them, they replied, "Well, we already knew that you were on the spectrum!" I am lucky to know people who have put up with my, sometimes erratic, social behaviour and still want to spend time with me.

I suffered in the work place. Looking back, I utterly loathed it. I became self-employed when I was quite young.

I now believe that a close family member suffered with the condition, acutely. They were treated throughout their life for many of the symptoms (depression, anxiety etc.) resulting from coping strategies. I now see that they were often confused, misunderstood and angry.

Undiagnosed individuals learn to survive. We have developed what seem to us to be reasonable coping strategies. 'Flight' being one in my repertoire, of which I am now very aware. Another widely employed strategy is alcohol consumption, often used as a short-term fix to 'anaesthetise' social anxieties. Many sufferers of drug addiction may well have undiagnosed ASD.

Others often see these strategies as rude or antisocial. I am so blessed to be with a partner who seems to understand many of these strategies and sees them for what they are. It still it makes me sad to know that my actions are sometimes upsetting and must test her patience. These self-taught strategies often lead to rejection, misinterpretation, loneliness, feelings of abandonment, anxiety, depression and so on.

I try to explain that what others do naturally often seems irrational and unnatural to me. Imagine going against what you feel is normal in order to be accepted in society. It is weird and draining.

I was so pleased and relieved to have a diagnosis. It explains so much. Although challenging, I am now replacing my self-taught coping strategies with more healthy ones."

Section 2
How we respond to unresolved issues

When we have unresolved issues, whether these are from the past or present, this creates conflict. Unresolved conflict needs addressing, otherwise it presents itself in unhealthy ways.

21. Addiction

When you are fighting with your emotions and want to get away from those feelings, you may turn to unhealthy behaviour or a substance to gain some temporary relief. The problem is that the emotions are still there and become more difficult to address the further you get sucked into addiction. Over time the emotions, stress and trauma you are trying to cover up, can appear heightened due to overuse of substances and the subsequent impact on you.

Cigarettes & vaping

When people come to me for help to give up cigarettes, I ask them why they believe they need to smoke. The most common response is to calm them down or to help with anxiety. I hear this often with clients, especially those who have been smoking for a decade or longer and fear the health risks. There is a great flaw with this thinking. The truth is cigarettes are more likely to cause anxiety. Smoking becomes another problem for you to overcome. If you do not experience this now, you will at some point.

The pull for smokers of cigarettes is the speed in which nicotine reaches the brain, which is approximately 10 seconds after the first puff. Initially the nicotine improves mood and reduces the feeling of stress. Many regular smokers do not finish their cigarettes, because they have had the 'hit' they desire. Whereas most social smokers do finish theirs because they are involved in the experience of smoking and are more likely to savour each drag of nicotine.

The problem arises for regular smokers because continued doses of nicotine results in changes in the brain chemistry.

This causes nicotine withdrawal symptoms whenever the supply of nicotine decreases. These withdrawal symptoms are similar to anxiety. Have you ever wondered how much of your anxiety is caused through smoking?

The logic in smoking to reduce anxiety is flawed because it actually creates anxiety. This is not only the anxiety from nicotine withdrawal but also from everything else that goes with being a smoker. You worry about how you smell to other people and what those individuals think of you as a smoker. You worry about needing a cigarette when you have not had one for a while. You might become anxious about your health and have fears that you will die a slow, painful and debilitating death from one of the dreadful diseases linked to smoking. Of course, you try to put this out of your mind because it is too unbearable to think about. Smoking gives you more things to worry about.

Take a moment to recall that first drag on a cigarette. The one when you take a big deep breath in. However, this time without a cigarette, take a big deep and slow breath into your belly, keeping your shoulders down and relaxed, then breathe out slowly. Do you notice how relaxing that is? Do another 10 of these deep breaths right now and observe how much calmer you feel. Focus on the breath, for those 10 breaths nothing else is important.

Now you have found an alternative way to naturally relax, needing nothing more than some air, your nostrils, lungs and a little bit of focus.

Nicotine can also be responsible for causing depression. Smoking stimulates the release of dopamine, which is a neurotransmitter in the brain. People who experience depression often have a low level of dopamine. Dopamine helps to create positive feelings. It also aids focus and concentration.

Once again, smoking influences the brain's natural processes causing the brain to switch off its own mechanism for making dopamine. Therefore, the supply of dopamine decreases between cigarettes. This would increase your desire to smoke. Someone who experiences depression needs to find other ways to stimulate the production of dopamine through natural methods. Creating a healthier lifestyle can help to achieve this.

Some people are moving away from cigarettes towards vapes in a bid to be healthier. Most vapes also contain nicotine. Behaviour around smoking vapes has changed for many smokers. Compared to cigarettes, people who vape reach for a puff more frequently.

There are deeply concerning health risks reported with vapes. Lung disease and deaths have been reported, as a consequence of vaping, to otherwise healthy people.

The idea of vaping as a replacement for cigarettes has never sat well with me. Let's keep it basic and logical. Our lungs are important organs for us to breathe in air so we can live. When you see what comes out of a vape and goes into someone's lungs, I find it hard to accept that vaping in any way can be okay and anything near a safe replacement for cigarettes.

There is a lot more to be learned about vaping but we know vapes contain chemicals, which are not natural substances for the body to process.

In summary smoking of any sort is likely to add to feelings of anxiety and depression in the long term. Most smokers want to stop at some point in their lifetime. Smoking is not a healthy or wise option to help you to feel better.

If you do decide to stop smoking, do so when the time feels right and you are ready to stop. You can seek help. When you stop smoking, the nicotine is out of your system in 48 hours – that is right, just 48 hours. Hypnotherapy is a great treatment for smoking and vaping cessation.

Cannabis & other drugs

Cannabis has many other names. The most common of those are marijuana and weed. Cannabis is sometimes used by anxiety or depression sufferers in a bid to 'escape' the feelings they want rid of.

Cannabis contains lots of different chemicals known as cannabinoids. Some examples are cannabidiol (CBD) and tetrahydrocannabinol (THC). THC is the main active ingredient in the cannabis plant and is illegal in many countries. Consuming THC will usually result in a high or sense of euphoria. CBD does not cause the same euphoric effects that occur with THC. CBD is used legally in many countries to help with a variety of health conditions.

Information on the serious health effects of other drugs is widely available. Some people are lucky and take drugs with no lasting effects and manage to get out before the addiction takes a strong hold but for many taking drugs can be life destroying.

Rather than go into the depths and science, I want to tell

you about some real-life experiences reported by my clients, following their experiences of taking cannabis and other drugs.

One man in his twenties was suffering from anxiety. The anxiety started on a night in which he smoked cannabis. This resulted in a severe panic attack when medics had to be called. This was his first ever panic attack and triggered longer term anxiety. The first panic attack was a severe trauma, which required healing. This was achieved by working with a combination of therapies. I have heard of this type of experience numerous times.

Another client of mine had taken MDMA (ecstasy) during a festival. They reacted badly as their view of everything became distorted. Longer term this resulted in a number of severe anxieties, including agoraphobia, fear of being on their own and fear of the being in the places where other panic attacks had happened. Often the anxiety escalates into other areas of life.

People rarely talk about the negative effects of cannabis. It tends to be thought of as a light or harmless social drug, which can be the case. However, for some people, taking cannabis can be a frightening experience. The same goes for other drugs. The message is simple. Do not take drugs because they could add to your problems and are certainly not a solution to mental or emotional challenges. The reality is they can create a variety of mental health problems and the experience can be very scary.

Alcohol

When does alcohol become a problem? This can be challenging to define but the following would provide a fair basis for concern:

- If you feel you need a drink.
- If you are using alcohol to hide stress, problems or feelings.
- If you are drinking alcohol secretly.
- If you are relying on alcohol to function.
- If you cannot go a day/evening without drinking.
- If your consumption is regularly over the recommended healthy allowance of units. At the time of writing, current advice is to drink no more than 14 units per week, which is the equivalent of 7 glasses or wine or 7 pints of beer or similar. It is recommended to have some alcohol-free days to enable the body to recover.

Just as with anything else you use to cover up feelings you are not wanting to feel or thoughts you do not want to think, in the long-term using alcohol makes you feel bad. You will wish you never started with it. Alcohol often results in people caring less about themselves and being unable to function. It is disempowering.

To feel better, it is important to address your emotions, problems and challenges you are facing in life. Also using techniques and tools for a more positive mindset become empowering. This results in taking control of the way you feel and your life without the need to rely on anything unhealthy or illegal to feel good.

If alcohol is a problem for you, make a start by cutting down. By all means seek help. As a therapist, if someone comes to me requesting help with alcohol, I want to understand the emotions and reasons behind it. We will then address the underlying issues because, once you resolve those, it becomes easier to feel more empowered and work towards not needing the substance.

Gambling

Gambling is another distraction and may come about through a gradual addiction. I have known guys gamble as a self-sabotage behaviour as well as for other reasons. If you gamble, you are wise enough to know that any win you are hoping for will be so rarely achieved and you will lose more money than you win. After all, gambling is a business and the business wins. However, gamblers are addicted to the feeling of anticipation.

It is that anticipation and rush of adrenalin which keeps gamblers hooked. Some people who gamble end up in absolute dire straits owing huge amounts of money and even stealing from friends and family. It is a vicious addiction and with its current internet availability is far too accessible.

That excitement whilst you wait, eagerly anticipating a win, gives you a high. You may win, very occasionally, but the reality is gambling will potentially destroy your life and the lives of those you love.

As with the other addictions, I have noted above, gambling will, in the long run, create more anxiety and stress than you may care to think about. In the end, it is not just you who suffers. Your family also pay the price, usually financially and certainly emotionally.

If you are gambling, I urge you to stop because it will not just drain your bank account but it will drain your mental and physical health. Gambling may be filling a hole in your life, which suggests something needs addressing. It may be used to cover up emotions, stresses and trauma. This too can be addressed. It may be a world you got sucked into unwittingly.

Whatever the reason, please seek help because gambling is another form of parasite which will leave damaging scars.

Porn and sex

I want to make it clear that I make no judgement on porn. What I am talking about here is when porn becomes addictive. Something that you 'need' and use to de-stress. If you are blotting out unwanted thoughts and feelings through porn or sexual activity, this is going to lead to suffering on your part and possibly on the part of those people close to you.

The other issue that can result from porn addiction is moving into child porn which, of course, is illegal. I have heard of cases which have gone to court where men in very responsible and trusting positions, e.g. psychiatrists and teachers, have gone to prison for downloading and sharing child porn. The reason they give is stress. Porn should not be used as a stress relief because potentially it can lead to more serious styles of porn, which cross the boundary into the underworld of criminal activity.

Whether you are actively engaging in child abuse or a viewer of child porn, you are participating in child abuse. Along with being morally wrong and heinous, it is against the law.

Sometimes when people feel bad about themselves, they revert to increased and unhealthy sexual activity. This may be having sex with numerous partners or taking unhealthy risks. If your behaviour has changed and fits this category, there are likely to be some deeper issues which need to be addressed.

As with other addictions, if you are using porn or sex as a means of hiding inner thoughts and feelings or to sabotage your own happiness, I encourage you to seek help before you regret it. As you seek riskier or more intense sexual behaviour, you may be putting yourself or others at risk in the long term through out of character and impulsive behaviour.

Food

Addiction to food is one of the most common addictions there is. The issue is how much of a problem it is for you and how does it impact your life? When people eat to cover up the way they feel, they are failing to address the underlying problems.

One problem with this addiction is that we need to eat food to live. With most, if not all, other addictions, we do not need them to survive so when we remove them from our lives they can be avoided completely. We cannot do this with food. This may be one reason why it is a challenging addiction to gain control over using will power alone and one that is easy to stray back into.

There are many reasons why people over-eat. Sometimes people eat through boredom, or food is used to fill a gaping hole in their lives. This may be related to someone they have lost or some area of unfulfillment. If you were sexually or physically abused, food may be used to create layers of protection, through fat, or to make yourself less desirable. This would be an unconscious response, meaning you are not aware that you are doing it for this reason.

Bear in mind the subconscious way of dealing with problems is not always logical. This means by trying to resolve one problem, it will sometimes create another problem. To resolve this, the initial problem (stress or trauma) requires healing and resolution.

You may have been deprived of food or types of food as a youngster and now are able to eat whatever you want. Whatever the reason behind over-eating, it may leave you feeling out of control and unable to be able to stop eating when you should.

These issues can be addressed so you can gain control. Very often when people address their diet, they also address other aspects of their lifestyle such as exercise, removing unnecessary stresses, alcohol consumption and other unhealthy behaviour. Many positives can come about through addressing emotional eating behaviour.

Ask yourself, "what are the feelings I am covering up?" Make a note of them so you can address these. Awareness is the first step to change.

Here are a few practical tips to help get your eating habits in a better balance.

- Ensure you eat mindfully; notice the taste and texture of the food you are eating.
- Do not skip breakfast because you will be more likely to eat unhealthily and more later in the day.
- Always eat sitting down and pay attention to each mouthful you take.
- Be aware of the taste and texture of the food.
- Eating a well-balanced diet will also help, because you feel better for getting the nutrients you need. It also becomes easier to recognise when your diet is slipping.

- Ensure you have protein with every meal.
- Mental health issues sometimes get in the way of looking after yourself, but you can buy in simple healthy foods or meals such as snack pots of fruit or nuts and seeds, well-balanced easy cook meals and pre-prepared salads.

Exercise

I pondered on whether to include exercise under this heading but some would say it can be an addiction. There is a good and bad side to exercise. For most people it is good. If you do have unhealthy reasons for exercising, in your heart of hearts you probably know it.

I have been keen on exercise since around the age of 12. In many ways, it created a great deal of balance in my life. It gave me a focus for channelling my attention into something positive together with reasons to eat well, look after myself and not drink alcohol.

Having exercise in your life provides many benefits, although it can have an addictive part to it. Anyone with an eating disorder could be addicted to exercise for all the wrong reasons. It is also easy to become addicted to the feel-good hormones released through exercise.

There are worse things to be addicted to than exercise. As long as you are healthy and remember to keep some balance in your life, please do enjoy your exercise.

Ensure you also have some downtime. A key aspect of exercising is including some recovery days. Your body heals and becomes stronger during these recovery phases. This can improve your fitness. Therefore, do not participate in hard or intense exercise every single day. Mix it around and have some days off.

Men suffering mental health issues can often find it helpful to exercise and can form good friendships through activity. So, on the whole, exercise is good. However, make time for other things such as friendships, relationships, relaxation and fun.

Summary

I raise these areas because we can often ignore the tools used to cover up our feelings. Awareness is the first step to change. Addictions can cause mental health issues but they are often used to cover up those feelings and thoughts you do not want. However, when you deal with the underlying issues, you are in a much better position to take charge of the addictive behaviour.

The relief you achieve from the addictive behaviour may appear good at the time but, in the long term, it becomes more damaging and will become a problem for you to add to the other issues which you were struggling with. If you recognise any of these signs please seek help.

22. Anxiety and panic attacks

Anxiety is a term used to describe a combination of symptoms related to feelings of fear or nervousness. Along with the physical symptoms common in anxiety, many people who suffer anxiety also worry a lot and experience many negative thoughts. They focus on the worst-case scenarios, which exacerbates the anxiety. Long-term anxiety can affect sleep, health and general well-being.

Anxiety comes in many forms but there are two basic types. The first is generalised anxiety or generalised anxiety disorder with the other type being specific anxiety.

Generalised anxiety disorder

Generalised anxiety disorder (GAD) is the term given to a condition whereby the sufferer experiences chronic worry and tension, thus causing high levels of stress. This term was introduced in 1980 when anxiety neurosis was split into GAD and panic disorder. GAD became a diagnostic classification in the third edition of the Diagnostic and Statistical Manual of Mental Disorders. Sufferers think of the worst-case scenarios, run these over and over in their minds and expect them to happen.

GAD can be all-consuming and stop people doing basic tasks such as going to the shops or holding down a job. GAD can be incredibly debilitating for some people and impact on every aspect of their lives. Other people can function, apparently, normally with GAD. In fact, many people sufferers associate with would not know they experienced anxiety.

Often GAD is experienced in individuals where:

- there is no specific event which triggered the anxiety.
- they may have had a parent/guardian who worried a lot or was depressed.
- they may have suffered birth trauma or other trauma at a very young age.
- they feel they have 'always' worried or suffered with anxiety.

Specific anxiety

I consider someone to have specific anxiety if they meet one or more of the following criteria:

- a specific event, or group of events, has triggered the anxiety.
- the person has not always suffered with anxiety.
- the person's anxiety is triggered in specific situations.

Does it matter which anxiety you have in terms of treatment?

It helps me, as a therapist, to understand the specific nature of a person's anxiety, even if it is of a more generalised type.

When someone suffers with GAD, there is a benefit in working with the subconscious mind to resolve any trauma and create positivity. However, teaching sufferers techniques is also important. I usually find those with GAD need more treatment than people with a more specific anxiety. It is also likely that they will always need to take care of their mental and emotional health, in the same way that someone with gastrointestinal issues has to take care of their digestive system on a long-term or permanent basis.

For anyone who has anxiety triggered by a specific event, it is beneficial to seek out and resolve the memory of that event held within the subconscious. It is also helpful to learn techniques that can be called upon instantly at any time.

Anxiety and depression

It is common for anxiety and depression to be experienced at the same time. They are both linked to the limbic system within the brain. Suffering from one of these challenges can set off the other.

Causes of anxiety

The root causes of anxiety can be very similar events to those which bring about depression, lack of confidence and other issues. Traumatic or stressful experiences can be a trigger. In the case of anxiety, those events will often cause us to experience feelings of fear, nervousness or panic. Along with this can come a lack of confidence, believing that you are not good enough and fear of being judged.

We usually feel isolated in these situations and appear not to hold the knowledge or skills to deal with it. You would have activated one of your innate survival responses, namely fight, flight or freeze. As this happens, we lock these memories into our subconscious.

Sometimes the causal events may, on the face of it, appear insignificant, especially if they happened when you were a youngster. However, at the time they were extremely traumatic or stressful. They may have left you feeling shocked, unsafe, helpless or had other possible responses, without the resources to deal with the situation or the knowledge to put it into a wider perspective. You could not access skills and knowledge which you held at the time. It is as if you shut down. The event, your perception of it and the feelings you had at the time were significant and left a lasting impression upon you.

Often anxiety is something that starts in childhood and continues into adulthood. However, events which happen to us in adulthood can also be the starting point for anxiety.

Think back to when the anxiety started for you. What was going on in your life? Can you recall that first trigger event or the series of stressful events which became too much? When you know the answers to these questions, you have the root causes. Once the root causes, and any associated information, are held within your subconscious mind, in its attempt to protect you and keep you safe, your mind will connect other events which may be "unsafe".

In terms of anxiety, the mind sees things as safe and unsafe. Anything which the mind portrays as unsafe will trigger anxiety. When I say "unsafe', I mean if the mind interprets any event as being a threat to you in terms of your overall safety. This will often be through a connection it has made to previous events in your life. In reality, most events which trigger anxiety are not a threat to our lives.

Examples of events which people might feel anxious about could be:

- Speaking in public.
- Being in a crowded room.
- People being sick.
- Answering the phone or door.

These are not anxieties we are born with. It is more likely that life events have triggered them through memory held within the subconscious mind. Let's look into this a little further:

The UDIN moment

Events which leave a lasting imprint on our subconscious minds, which were at the time shocking, traumatic or stressful, are UDIN events.

U = Unexpected – the event was unexpected. A shock. Not planned for.

D = Dramatic – you were unprepared and therefore the event had a powerful impact on you. It caused cellular and chemical changes within you very quickly, changing your energy, physicality and emotional balance.

I = Isolating – in that moment you feel alone. You need someone to give you a big hug and say "it's okay, you are safe, I am here for you" but it does not happen. If it does happen, consciousness might have shut down before so it is no help.

N = No strategy or resources – you were unprepared for this event and in that moment were unable to access the knowledge, wisdom or skills to overcome it. You are effectively stuck in that moment.

When you experience a UDIN moment, the mind stores a variety of information. This data could be things you see consciously and unconsciously at the time, related to smells, feelings and sensations, sounds and sometimes taste related. I have known people to experience a shocking moment at a meal-time which can cause anxiety around certain foods.

In future, if your mind recognises a situation as being similar to your UDIN moment, it will put you on alert, into the fight or flight response, even freeze response, in order to protect you. It wants you to know there is danger. In reality, the (perceived) danger is rarely real.

What an incredible safety system we have. The problem is, in terms of anxiety, it is usually too sensitive or you could say it responds to current and future events based on old information which no longer represents the person you are, including your skills, knowledge, wisdom and capabilities.

Let me give you some examples:

Event 1: childhood

You are at school and put your hand up very eagerly to answer a question in class. The teacher offers for you to respond with your answer. Unfortunately, you get the answer wrong. The entire class laughs at you. Your cheeks go bright red and, in that moment, you want to shrivel up into a ball or run away but you cannot.

This is what happened

In that moment your limbic system kicked into action and you accessed your natural survival response of fight, flight or freeze. As far as your brain and body were concerned, you were under attack. You would have been flushed with stress hormones, your digestion shut down, you could not think clearly and other processes of the fight, flight or freeze response kicked in.

Belief

In that moment, you would have formed a belief. An example would be "it is not safe to speak up" or "I must not be centre of attention". You then spend the rest of your life doing your best to avoid situations which would put you in a similar situation.

Future

You will experience anxious thoughts and feelings at the possibility of being centre of attention. Whenever you go into a situation similar to this, i.e. speaking in public or being centre of attention, your limbic system, because it wants to protect you, will kick in. You will go into the fight, flight or freeze response. This is your body's natural attempt to 'keep you safe'.

Reality

You were absolutely safe. You were under no actual threat to your life or about to come to any harm. However, remember, our physical make-up is still that of our ancestry, ready to fight or run like our life depends on it from that sabre-toothed tiger or to go into the freeze response to preserve life.

Truth

You were not under any threat. You were safe. Getting a question wrong is all part of life's learning and we all get things wrong at some time or another. That is how we develop and grow. The children were either cruel or perhaps naïve and immature to laugh.

Understanding

As an adult you would probably look back at this event and think, "that cannot be the reason I hate being centre of attention. Surely the anxiety did not start because of that event." You find it hard now, with all your life experience, to believe that this could have been a trigger. However, this is an example of an event which could trigger anxiety, lack of confidence, fear of public speaking, fear of being centre of attention and other restrictive issues.

Event 2: adulthood

You are at work and the boss informs you that you have made a big mistake in your work that has gone out to a client.

This is what happened

Once again, in that moment your limbic system kicked into action and you accessed your natural survival response of fight, flight or freeze. Your thoughts are clouded, your heart is beating fast, your breathing rate increases and your stomach knots up.

Belief

In that moment, you would have formed a belief. An example would be "I will get fired, have no money and could lose my house" or "I am incompetent". You will be running through all the possible worst-case scenarios from the impact of this situation.

Future

From now on you will most likely have a lot of self-doubt and check your work over and over. You may change career as you believe you are not cut out for that type of work or the stress of it. You feel less confident in situations you previously handled easily.

Reality

Your boss had not indicated that you would get fired. The reality is that a phone call is made to the client explaining the error and the situation is put to bed. The boss appreciated that this was an out of character error. Procedures were put in place to ensure it did not happen again. However, as far as your limbic system is concerned you were experiencing a threat to your life. The trauma has already occurred and the memory is stored.

Truth

You were absolutely safe. You were under no actual threat to your life or about to come to any harm. You were not fired and all the worst-case scenarios did not come to fruition. Life continues as normal except for your own thoughts, worries and emotions.

Understanding

Your logical mind would probably say that all is fine and nothing has changed but you struggle to get that UDIN moment out of your mind and the possible impact it could have had on your life. You now live in fear of making another mistake. This is because your limbic system is doing its good work trying to 'keep you safe'. It has started a programme running, related to this event, which causes you to feel anxious in similar situations. This serves as a red flag warning system.

Fight, flight and freeze responses

The most common symptoms of the fight or flight response are:

- shallow breathing, which may lead to hyperventilation
- heart racing
- clammy hands
- perspiring
- clouded thinking
- digestion shuts down
- more blood and oxygen goes to working muscles
- shaking
- limited blood flow to extremities results in a feeling of cold or tingling
- dilated pupils
- nausea

Fight, flight or freeze

All three responses relate to stress and trauma and are triggered by our natural inbuilt security system, known as the limbic system. This is because the brain is aware of a perceived harmful event or believes there is a threat to your survival.

We are born with only two fears: the fear of falling and the fear of loud noises. This means that anything else we fear is usually the result of events which happen in life. The first sign of snow and the shops sell out of the basics because we go back into our ancestral survival pattern. We worry there will not be sufficient provisions, even though many of us have chest freezers and kitchen cupboards stocked up with enough food for the next three months.

Just as when man lived in caves, we still have a need for survival, but we apply this to modern day worries such as financial problems, relationships, work and family. When we are over-focused on potential problems, we activate our fear response, also known as the fight or flight response, which is based on a primeval reflex. In this response we only have two options (1) to stand up and fight for our cause; or (2) to run away from the situation.

In this state, our body is preparing for action, which is why the physical changes occur. Stress hormones are released as more blood is being pumped to the working muscles and less blood is being pumped towards areas such as digestion, our breathing prepares with increased speed and becomes shallower and our heart races. We are ready for action.

There is a problem though. Whereas physically we are geared up to run or fight, in modern society, we can rarely do either of these which holds us in this 'ready for action' state. We are therefore holding onto the stress. Doing this long term impacts our well-being.

We can activate our fight or flight response in completely unthreatening situations, such as being in a traffic jam causing us to be late for an appointment, arguing with someone because they jumped a queue, having to stand up and talk in public or attending a social gathering.

The response is the same as it was centuries ago but we are limited in our use of the fight or flight response. For example, you cannot punch that person who jumped the queue. Well, you could, but you would probably be arrested and I certainly would not recommend it. You cannot run from the traffic jam or get out of that social event. Therefore, you are stuck. Stress causes us to be stuck in a response which was designed to last seconds or, at the most, a couple of minutes. If the response continues to build, then the result could be a panic attack, which is a very unpleasant out-of-control feeling as you struggle to bring your breathing under control.

We have an alternative, which is the freeze response. The freeze response is another part of our physical structure which also links back to our ancestry. When the tiger had cornered us and was about to devour us, our brain had assessed the situation and decided there was only one option remaining because we could not run away or fight. We had to initiate the freeze response. When you activate this response, you have run out of all other options. There is no opportunity to run or fight, you feel helpless and hopeless. You are in serious danger. "I cannot run or fight, I must therefore freeze or die." It has become apparent over recent years that by not releasing the freeze response this causes us to hold on to trauma.

It is highly unlikely we will get attacked by a wild animal in this modern day unless we put ourselves in danger's way, yet this natural instinct to freeze is ingrained in us. Therefore, we apply the freeze response to situations which are stressful. Some of which may be serious or dangerous.

Usually, the freeze response happens in more seriously traumatic events such as being threatened with a weapon, being involved in an accident or being sexually abused or raped. However, it can happen in what appear to be less serious events, if at the time you have no option to flee the situation or fight, such as a teacher telling you off as a child or being bullied. The brain decides there is only one option remaining, which is to go into the freeze response. You are most likely unaware of the freeze as consciousness appears to shut down.

In the freeze response you go into a self-paralysis protection mode. You become physically, mentally and emotionally immobilised, which results in you consciously being unable to feel or experience the distressing event. This is our innate protection mode. Perhaps you can recall an event when you felt you could not move or speak. It is only after the event you consider how you could have dealt with it.

In the freeze response, effectively you hold the trauma because humans do not automatically discharge the freeze response. This can cause psychological, emotional and physical challenges following the harrowing incident. Often this is referred to as Post Traumatic Stress Disorder or PTSD.

Wild animals discharge the freeze response as soon as possible after the incident. If you wish to see this, I suggest you conduct an internet search for "animal release of freeze response". It is quite an amazing natural process to view. I must warn you prior to watching, it is not the most pleasant thing to view but once the freeze response has been released, the animal has let go of the trauma and can go about its business.

Discharging the freeze response releases trauma. If we did the same as wild animals, we would not have so many fears or inhibitions. This is one example of how amazing the mind and body are when nature takes its true course.

Because we are so domesticated, we do not usually discharge the freeze response and therefore stay stuck in the trauma. This means we develop fears and phobias and may struggle to deal with certain situations.

These traumas need to be released in order to free you. I would only ever recommend dealing with such situations under the guidance of a suitably qualified therapist. Someone who works with the subconscious mind such as a hypnotherapist or a practitioner of Emotional Freedom Technique or Matrix Reimprinting. Of course, if you believe any other appropriate therapy works well for you, then go with it.

Summary

In terms of anxiety, you can recognise that it is a natural response, linked back to the way we are put together. We hold trauma within our subconscious mind. The information is activated through the limbic system. However, that trauma can be released resulting in freedom from many of the challenges you are facing.

Here is a quick look at how it all comes together:

The process in a nutshell

Information comes into the brain
↓
That information is processed by the brain
↓
Information is Interpreted as safe/unsafe
(this may be based on previous events/information already stored)
↓
Depending on whether the interpretation is considered positive or negative, or safe or unsafe, the stress response, also known as the fight, flight or freeze response, may be triggered.

You could say that, whether you suffer anxiety or other mental health issues, this is most likely based on 'information' entering our subconscious and stored there, but not necessarily coming into our conscious awareness. The data is processed through the mind and body. Based on a very brief subconscious analysis of a current or future situation, we revert to the old stored information and decide how 'safe' the current or future event is. In effect, our response becomes a programmed response.

You can try to make conscious sense of the situation and tell yourself that you are being ridiculous or that all is okay but if the programme you are running is based on old information and stored in that subconscious mind then conscious sense makes little or no difference.

An example of this is someone who has a fear of flying. Some people who have the fear may have had a previous experience when flying which they found scary. At the time of the UDIN moment, they formed a belief which is 'flying is dangerous', despite the fact they landed safely. This is the memory stored in the subconscious mind as a constant reminder that flying is dangerous. In order to release the fear, releasing the memory and any emotion linked to it has proven to be hugely beneficial.

Panic attacks

Panic attacks can occur suddenly and unexpectedly or happen after a period of anxiety. When triggered suddenly this may be because your subconscious mind recognises a 'perceived' threat based on all the information stored in your subconscious mind. You may not know why you are experiencing a panic attack, which can make it even more stressful.

Some people awaken after a night's sleep straight into a panic attack. Most panic attacks last less than 10 minutes but can last up to an hour. Some people will believe they are having a heart attack because of the intense nature of a panic attack.

If you suffer regular panic attacks, you may be diagnosed with panic disorder. People suffering from panic disorder will have feelings of anxiety and panic regularly. These can happen at any time and often for no obvious reason.

The symptoms of a panic attack are similar to those of anxiety, although more severe. Added to these, there is a strong sense of terror and loss of control. It becomes incredibly difficult to catch your breath, which can result in feeling dizzy or faint. It can feel as if the walls are closing in. Panic attacks can be quite a surreal experience.

Many people who suffer anxiety will fear having a panic attack, even if they have never had one before. This keeps them stuck in anxiety and fear.

If you suffer with panic attacks, it is useful for your partner, or anyone else you feel appropriate, to be prepared so they can assist you and provide reassurance. Here are some tips for that person if they are in a position help:

- Be a calming influence.
- Ensure they are not bent over or in any way obstructing their breathing. They need to sit or stand upright.
- Do not get too close to them. Give them some space. They will feel they need air.
- They may want a window opened.
- Ensure they are in a safe place and remove anything that may be causing stress.
- Do not ask them questions. They may not be able to talk and may not know why they are having the panic attack.
- Ask them to mirror your breathing whilst placing one of their hands on their heart or across their forehead – do the same as it helps them to mirror what you do. Breathe in slowly through your nose and out through your mouth. By mirroring you, this also gives them some focus away from the panic.
- Have some water available in case they wish to have some. Suggest to them that they sip the water. If they were to gulp the water, it may cause them to lose their breath.
- Give them a ball, apple or orange (or other object if necessary) and ask them to move it from hand to hand. This can be a useful distraction technique.
- If what you are doing is not working, consider seeking medical intervention.

Overcoming anxiety

Every person is different but in general I have found a combination of techniques to address the conscious analytical mind together with working through the information held within the subconscious mind to achieve impressive results when addressing anxiety and panic attacks.

Accessing and addressing the information stored in the subconscious mind and releasing the emotions is the most powerful way of creating change. The subconscious mind is very pliable, in that it will adapt easily to new and positive information. For these reasons, I favour subconscious and energy therapies over conscious therapy.

Conscious therapy, e.g. talking and exploring behaviours and emotions, may help you make sense of your response and any involvement from other people but the subconscious programme is often still running.

You can find more specific information and help for anxiety in my book, 'The Energy of Anxiety'.

23. Grief

Grief is something we all go through in life. When I look back at the many bereavements of family members throughout my life, I have recollections of the men in the family always being stoic. They would fill the role of being the prop for the rest of the family. The man would get on and do any necessary organising and sort out paperwork and such like. They would be strong and solid, following tradition and protocol.

Considering the clients I have worked with who sought help for a variety of issues (e.g. weight loss, depression and addiction), sometimes we worked to release the emotions attached to bereavement. You are probably wondering how I ended up helping people to release grief when this was often not their reason for contacting me. This is because although they came to me to address their over-eating behaviour, health issues, depression, anxiety or addiction, behind the problem was grief. They were not always aware of this when they booked their session.

I expect that over the decades and centuries, men have been experiencing grief and covering it up through unhealthy behaviour. Alternatively, it comes out in some other way through their mental or physical health.

Unprocessed grief is another suppressed emotion. Grief reveals itself and sometimes not in the most obvious way.

When it comes to grief, it is important to feel safe so you can let your emotions out. When my dad died, I decided that I would take my own advice and let emotions flow. This enabled me to move more swiftly through the grieving process.

Stresses of Modern Man

Even so, grief can hit you at any time. If grief strikes me, it is usually when I am riding my bicycle on my own. I could be thinking about anything, perhaps a memory or another person, and then I experience the grief, and the emotion flows. I never see this as a bad thing. It is normal to get reminders and sometimes they come at unexpected moments. My message to you is, let the emotions flow. If you need to cry, then cry. If men were not meant to cry, they would not have tear ducts.

There is a plethora of symptoms attached to grief. Each of us experience grief in our own way. Whatever you are experiencing, please do not judge yourself. There is no right or wrong to grief.

Here are some symptoms you may have experienced:

- Crying, sometimes overwhelmingly
- Stress
- Depression
- Headaches and migraines
- Difficulty sleeping
- Increased appetite
- Feelings of detachment
- Isolation from friends and family
- Irrational behaviour
- Worry and anxiety
- Frustration and anger
- Guilt
- Fatigue
- Loss of appetite
- Aches and pains
- Health issues

Do not judge yourself for the way you handle death. My dad did not cry when his mother passed but did when his rescue dog died. Allow any emotions to flow. Pushing them away will only cause them to come out in another way which is likely to be less healthy.

Life is complicated and this often results in death being complicated too, for a variety of reasons.

Parental death

The hardest death we are all likely to experience is the death of a parent. If you had a wonderful relationship with your parent then this will naturally create a gaping hole in your life. Some people are so close to a parent they have no idea how they will function without them in the future. This can create anxiety amongst other emotions.

On the other side of this are those difficult relationships with a parent. I struggled with my dad at times. What I realised, sometime after this death, was that, in many ways, we were similar. This is not necessarily an easy thing to admit when a relationship feels strained, but it helped me understand why I found him challenging.

For some, the relationship with a parent is damaged beyond repair, leaving you estranged. When you receive the phone call which tells you they have gone, you have no idea how to react. How do you process such information and what do you do next? These are questions which run through your mind.

When I talk about a parent, this is not always one of two people who procreated you. This is the person who brought you up, and treated you as their own child. Your bond with this person is as strong as it would be if they were your own blood parent.

If you have suffered abuse from this person, this can result in a plethora of emotions. Or perhaps in some other way your upbringing was massively dysfunctional, maybe through drugs or alcohol. If there was not an appropriate parent and child relationship, death of a parent can leave you feeling quite hollow. It is as if a part of you believes you should be grieving but the emotion is blank.

Sometimes those emotions come but after a period of time, once you have moved through the various stages of bereavement.

As I said, relationships are complicated. Death of a parent, can be one of the hardest to deal with. Accept whatever you are feeling. There is no right or wrong.

Death of a child

I have always believed that losing a child is not something anyone should have to go through. However, sadly this happens and for many reasons. The depth of emotional pain experienced through the loss of a child is unimaginable for most of us.

The healing process is slow. You may ask "can it ever be healed?". The truth is, I do not know if full healing can take place. This probably depends largely on your beliefs. If you have faith or a spiritual connection, then you may well be able to take great comfort in this. I certainly find spirituality has given me a very helpful foundation for many of life's experiences.

Depending on the circumstances of a child's death, people often find comfort in charity work. Some set up a foundation in their memory to create a positive and lasting legacy. Others will set about getting a law changed in Parliament if relevant to the circumstances of their death. Someone else may turn to creativity, such as writing music or a book. I am of the view that if something helps, then go with it. There is no one-size-fits-all in grief.

Death of a spouse or partner

Losing a partner can happen at any time. The circumstances of the loss impact on how you grieve. When it happens unexpectedly, there is the initial shock. It can take months to come to a realisation that you are not living in some sort of nightmare. Life can feel rather surreal. Usually, people rally around you initially but things can become tough when those people get back to their normal lives and you are left with the vast hole to fill.

Being in a relationship also usually means a split of responsibilities. Good relationships play to each other's strengths. If this is the case, you need to pick up the other half of responsibilities. You may need to seek help either from professionals, for example, for any financial issues, or from friends or other service providers if you do not feel able to take on some tasks.

If you have young children, there is an entire family in grief. You need to deal with life's day-to-day tasks and create some sort of routine. Do not be afraid to ask for help.

Along with the grief, you must deal with the silence. Waking up in the morning on your own can be hard to bear too. There can be a lot of loneliness. Some people cope with being on their own fine. Others need company of some sort. This might be when you get a dog or cat. You might volunteer for a charity or get a part-time job. You may take up a hobby or do some walking. Just to see other people walking around can help you feel part of a community. There are lots of ways to have social interaction, which is a basic human need. Even introverts need some level of social connection if only for brief periods of time.

Death of a friend

Losing a close friend can be as hard, and sometimes harder, than losing a relative. It all depends on the relationship you had with them and the circumstances of their death. When you lose someone who is considered too young to die, this can leave you with a mix of emotions. When you lose that friend, you have had for forty years or the one who suffered, or has left a young family, there is such a feeling of unfairness.

Sometimes you gain comfort in providing support for their family. You might do a reading at their funeral. Of course, you also have wonderful memories.

Your beloved pet

We build powerful bonds with our pets. The love we have for them is linked with a feeling of responsibility. For many of us, a pet is a member of the family. We often refer to ourselves as mummy and daddy when we talk to our pets. How we communicate with our pets is different to humans but we still talk to them and form a unique and special bond. You are allowed to feel grief for the loss of a beloved pet. Just as with humans, sometimes we lose a pet in a tragic way. Again, you will need to heal.

Sometimes we have to decide to euthanise our pet to stop any suffering but this can cause us to believe we are responsible for their death. You may question whether you made the right decision or if you did it at the right time. As long as your decision is from a place of love, the very same love you have always held for your darling pet, then you made the right decision. If you are questioning whether you did this, I am sure you did.

I take great comfort when I lose a beloved pet that I gave them a loving home. I cared for them in the very best way I could and they knew, beyond doubt, that I loved and adored them. That is the deal, right? An unconditional love between you both. So much love that you were prepared to break your own heart to stop their suffering. You did the right thing.

It is likely that a man would want to cover up those emotions. Telling himself "I shouldn't be feeling like this, it was just an animal". Not at all. It was a living being which you had a strong bond and deep love for. Allow yourself to go through the grieving process for your beloved pet. Anyone who does not agree with this does not understand the strength of that bond.

Feelings, emotions and more

The death of a loved one can be complicated. Along with the grief can come a bag of other emotions. You could experience any of the following:

- Regret

- Guilt
- Helplessness
- Anger
- Anxiety
- Depression
- Denial

Let's look at these in turn:

Regret

Regret is a common feeling after losing a loved one. Relationships are complicated. However, in life there is only one thing we can do and that is our best. Following the death of a loved one, we may decide that our best was not good enough. Some people believe they should have seen them more often or helped them more. Perhaps you feel regret because you were not on good terms with them when they died. Perhaps you missed years of their life for different reasons.

Everything I have noted above are normal reactions to the death of a loved one. As I mentioned, we do our best. Our best is based on so many things. However, it does not include what someone else does. Our best is not what society expects. It is not our ideal view of how everything should be.

Reality is we do not live in a fairy tale. Life throws all sorts at us throughout our lives. This affects the way we live our life, our emotions, belief system, personality, behaviour, relationships, health and many other aspects. Therefore, when I talk about doing our best, this is based on all of this and more. Our best may be distancing ourselves; it may be trusting them to make their own decisions about their health, it may be being angry with them. All of this is how humans over the centuries have functioned. You are no different.

Therefore, you did your best, given the complexities of life. There is no one-size-fits-all. There is no perfect way to be. When someone close to you has passed over, your life has changed. How you view things can change in an instant. So, when you have regrets, you are having these from a different standpoint. We cannot judge what we did in the past based on what we know now. If we do this, we are creating a false reality.

We have to consider your entire relationship with this person, not just what happened in those final weeks, days or hours. We experience regret over the things we cannot change. What point is regret if we cannot change something? Regret creates personal suffering. It is self-punishment. It is drinking a little poison every day to make yourself feel bad.

You did nothing bad. You did your best. Accept that life is complicated, as are relationships, and dying is a part of life, the finality of life that every single person can say with surety they will experience. What is the sense in regretting whatever part you did or did not play in that person's life? They are at peace. There is no need for you to be inflicting emotional pain upon yourself. That would be a waste of your life.

Trust that you are a good person. I know this because people generally are good. Sometimes good people make mistakes or show their emotional pain in a way that hurts others but they are still good people. Appreciate you have always done your best, based on your own circumstances, emotions and experiences.

Guilt

Guilt can be similar to regret. In fact, guilt often happens because of regret. Everything I have said about regret holds true for guilt. Guilt is also a very over-used emotion in everyday life. Guilt is at the core of Roman Catholicism. It keeps people in check and under control. Just to be clear, I am not getting into a debate on religion, that is far beyond the scope of this book and I hold no issue with Catholics.

I have witnessed people experiencing guilt way beyond anything they should be feeling. One of my clients attended a Catholic school. Although not a practicing Catholic, the preachings of the school resulted in a strong obsessive-compulsive disorder for my client, which continued through into adulthood. Through our sessions they were able to overcome this.

I also believe guilt is something which can be passed down to us, almost as if it is in our DNA. I have witnessed far too many honourable people experiencing high levels of guilt. Some people have it ingrained in them to apologise for nearly everything they say and do.

I ask, "what use is guilt?" I struggle to find a great use for it other than to stop us punching someone in the face or shooting them as we walk down the High Street because we dislike their face.

Guilt is another form of self-punishment. Continuing to sip from the poisonous cup, enough to cause you pain and discomfort. Enough to stop you enjoying life.

Following the death of someone close, guilt often causes

people to believe they had greater responsibility than they did. You start thinking that you should have done certain things whilst they were alive.

We are here on earth for several reasons, one of which is to enjoy life. Guilt stops you from enjoying life to the full. You might enjoy moments of life but not as much as you should. Guilt would never allow you to fully enjoy life. It's a nag in the background. Guilt can also cause self-sabotaging behaviour just to make sure you never live a happy and fulfilled life.

Do you believe that this person who you are grieving for would have wanted you to feel guilt and to live a life based on such an emotion? Definitely not and, if they did, then their own personal set of beliefs would be sadly misaligned.

As I have said, most people in life are good. I am sure you are one of them. Ask yourself, "what purpose does guilt serve?" If it is also to punish you, then acknowledge that you have done your best. You did all you could have, given everything that went before.

Given the complexities of life, you have done your best. Let it go.

Helpless

There are many situations in which a loved one dies which links to those left behind feeling helpless. When we feel helpless, we believe we needed to do more but the reality is there was no more for you to do.

We all play our roles in the lives of others. You played your role in this person's life, whether you are a father, son, friend, colleague or whatever part you played. You were not supposed to be their saviour too. They did not need to be saved. Whatever their age, they lived their full life, whatever that entailed. They passed over to peace and are now resting. The person not at peace is you.

The feelings we experience come with our own expectations. We all want life to be a fairy tale. However, the reality is life is not all joy and happiness. There are also challenges. It helps to see the tough experiences in life as opportunities for us either to grow and develop from or to let go of. Perhaps your challenge is to let go of needing to be the saviour and accepting that life is not eternal because, on a more soulful level, we chose it to be that way.

Anger

Anger is part of the grieving process for some people. It can be directed at many different people, including yourself, the person who has died, the medical team taking care of them, other members of the family or life itself.

It is not uncommon to feel anger towards the person who has died. How dare they die and leave you to carry on? The truth is they died because they knew you could carry on without them. It was just you who has yet to discover this. They have done all they came into this world to do whether they died an old person or a young person. This is a more spiritual take on the situation but gaining fresh perspectives can be beneficial in moving through the grieving process.

Anger also suggests that something was wrong. Just as with the other emotions, when you are saying something is wrong you are once again coming from an ideological point of view.

Humans have been on earth for billions of years, yet we are still unwilling to accept that life is not perfect.

Some people shift from anger into acceptance of the situation. The way they may do this is to become pro-active. This helps occupy their mind and give them the feeling of purpose and hope. Their energy becomes more positive. This may be a way of channelling the pain they are feeling, especially if the loss was shocking or traumatic.

Ways to direct that positivity may be to help create a new law. For example, if you need to highlight that a drug used was dangerous then put your energies into that. Some people set up charities or get involved with one that has already formed. Taking action to create something of benefit to others in that person's memory can be a productive way to heal.

Anxiety

Anxiety often happens years before someone close to you dies. People are anxious about losing that person. Frequently this relates to a parent, especially with the awareness that they are ageing or their health is not so good. Someone who has always been there for you, who can be called upon at any time with your concerns and worries, with the knowledge they will support you. There is a fear of losing that powerful connection.

There can be a fear and dread of going on without them. However, when death does happen, you realise you can go on, taking each day at a time. There will be moments when you want them by your side or you want to call them. This is natural, especially when you might want to ask them something or tell them about something you have achieved.

You can connect with them and you may believe at times they are reminding you that they are still with you, just not in a physical structure. When I leave my work studio at the rear of my garden on an evening and look up at the night sky, I often see a star twinkling back at me. This is my dad. Some people see a robin redbreast and know that is a loved one come to see them. Visiting their place of rest or connecting with some sort of memento or a photo can bring comfort.

We lose people and pets in the form we know them but they always leave a lasting imprint on our heart.

Depression

More people than realise suffer from depression following the loss of a loved one. It is common not to make that connection. Death is rarely straightforward and the specific reasons behind the depression may vary hugely.

Depression could set in because of a feeling you have about yourself. This might relate to some situations I have covered already. You may feel you failed to do enough for that person or perhaps you were not there when they died. Depression sets in with a feeling of hopelessness or helplessness.

You may regret the argument you had and then did not see them for two years. These situations and others can cause you to hold those negative feelings.

You may feel overwhelmed by the many things you need to sort out following their death. You may be the one to sort out the Will and documentation, clear the house or help out another relative. This might feel like an enormous responsibility. These situations can also result in depression.

Another common reason for depression is, quite simply, the loss of that person. I have known many clients say how losing someone has left a hole in their heart.

Depression does not necessarily set in immediately. It can be many months later before you realise that you feel so down. This could be why many people do not make the connection between bereavement and depression.

Denial

Denial is a way of surviving the loss of someone and this may be experienced prior to their death. This could be when you receive the bad news that someone you are close to is terminally ill or has had a terrible accident.

In denial, you block out the emotions you are not ready to feel. You try to continue with life as you know it. In denial you appear more able to deal with the practicalities. You probably keep yourself very busy and do not want to face the reality of the situation.

The emotions you are blocking out will be suppressed. You go numb. However, those emotions will not have disappeared forever. Denial delays the grieving process. It paces you through grief at a rate which is more manageable.

As you begin to accept your loss, you start the process of healing. As this happens those suppressed feelings will rise to the surface. This can be a surprise to some people as they wonder why they are feeling so emotional months or years after their loss. The reason is those emotions were always there but not ready to be expressed.

Beliefs and life changes

Losing a loved one can cause you to reflect on life. You may make some big life changes as you reflect upon your own situation. I have known people to take action regarding their own health and well-being. It may cause you to face the finality of life and therefore look at your own existence. You may ask yourself some questions:

- Am I living the life I want?
- Am I procrastinating?
- Am I looking after myself?
- Am I achieving the goals I have set myself?
- Am I happy?
- How can I make my life better?

You might start to make changes. Perhaps you decide to stop smoking, lose weight or become more active. You may decide to change career or move house to somewhere you have desired to live for some time. Through death of a loved one, we can learn and grow. Perhaps their passing gift to you is to give you the kick up the backside you needed to improve your own life.

You might decide to take a more spiritual path. This can help you see life and death in a brighter light. You may ponder on whether we have a soul. Does that soul continue after death? In which case it is only the physical body which has passed. The soul goes on and continues through into another life once the lessons from the life just experienced have been integrated.

It comforts me to believe that life is an experience and we are here to learn to develop. We leave this earth when we have completed all we came here to do, whatever our age when we die. There is more to explore in terms of spirituality. For the purpose of this book, I shall whet your appetite and leave it here.

In summary

When you know that the death of a loved one is imminent, you may believe you are prepared for the inevitable. However, as prepared as you believe you are, when it happens it still hits you hard. There is still a feeling of shock, whatever the circumstances. For a while, it seems as if you are living a surreal existence. Someone once in your life never to be there again. This takes time to heal.

Go gently and do not disregard your emotions. Do not feel you have to sort everything. Get help where you can. You do not have to do everything immediately. There are no hard and fast rules when it comes to grief. Do what feels right for you. Remember that whatever that is, and however you handle the situation, you are doing your best. Most importantly, be kind to yourself.

24. Insomnia

Humans have a natural sleep cycle which is part of our circadian rhythm. This is an internal process which regulates the sleep-wake cycle throughout each 24-hour period. Put another way, it is our internal clock, which knows when to awaken and when to sleep. When this works smoothly, we should fall asleep easily, have a quality night's sleep and feel re-energised in the morning.

Sleep is fundamental to our well-being. Insomnia may involve struggling to get off to sleep, waking up throughout the night and drifting in and out of consciousness or falling to sleep but waking up some hours later and failing to get back to sleep.

There is usually a precursor or root cause to insomnia. Often this is stress related, which can come in many forms, including anxiety. When you are mentally in stress, this will also create stress within the physical body. We must acknowledge the connection between mind and body.

In stress, the body is creating additional stress hormones such as adrenalin and cortisol. This keeps you in the sympathetic nervous system, i.e. the stress system. When it is time to rest, your body needs to be in the parasympathetic nervous system, also known as the rest and digest phase. Stress can limit your time in this phase or stop you reaching it altogether.

Many people with anxiety issues also have gastrointestinal issues such as irritable bowel syndrome. This is because they are not reaching the rest and digest phase when the body will naturally relax and digest food.

Your immune system releases a small protein called cytokines. These help the body fight inflammation and infection and are key in recovery from illness and injury. When the body is deprived of sleep, it may decrease production of these protective cytokines. Therefore, when you lack sleep, it takes so much longer to recover from both injury and illness.

The hormonal status of the body changes during sleep. Melatonin levels increase at night-time, which helps you to feel sleepy. However, some people have a melatonin deficiency, which can disrupt sleep. This deficiency may be long term or triggered through bouts of stress.

The sleep process is a very specific and intelligent system of the body and mind. Typically, a person would begin a sleep cycle every 90-120 minutes. Therefore, during a night, you would expect to have four to five sleep cycles which run smoothly and concurrently.

There are two key aspects of the sleep cycle known as rapid eye movement (REM) and non-REM sleep. There are four stages to non-REM sleep, which occur prior to REM sleep.

The first stage of non-REM sleep is the period when you are drifting off to asleep. You are probably familiar with this stage of sleep as it is easy to be disrupted and revert to a waking state in this phase. Some people experience muscle contractions which jerk them awake during this phase. These are called hypnic or hypnagogic jerks.

In stage two, you are in a light sleep. The brain produces sudden increases in brain wave frequency known as sleep spindles. The brain waves slow down. During this phase the heart rate and breathing regulate and body temperature drops.

If you are someone who likes to nap during the day, you should only be napping during the first two phases. This would be for approximately 20 minutes. Otherwise moving into the next stages, outside of your key sleep period, can affect the quality of your night-time sleep.

The third and fourth stages are deep sleep. During these phases there is no eye movement or muscle activity. You would be less likely to be awoken than during any of the other stages. Deep sleep is the most restorative and restful period of sleep. It is essential for mind and body to recover and rejuvenate.

As you sleep, the levels of stress hormones decrease and then rise again as your body prepares to awaken. However, if you are run down, these levels do not rise as they should when you awaken. This causes you to feel needy of more sleep.

From deep sleep you move into REM, which often occurs 90 minutes following commencement of sleep, although can happen at any point. During REM sleep we dream and our eyes move rapidly. Brain waves status is similar to that experienced during wakefulness. Our breathing rate increases. The body goes into a state of paralysis whilst dreaming.

Dreams are a method of processing information. As strange as some dreams are, they represent data stored in the subconscious mind. Sometimes this may relate to a television programme you were watching, a person you saw recently or challenges you are facing in life. Dreaming is the mind doing its own processing and filing. The length of REM periods increase as the night continues.

The cycle then repeats itself, but with each cycle you spend less time in the deeper stages of sleep and more time in REM sleep.

I am sure you appreciate just how crucial regular quality sleep is to feeling good. Without quality sleep your mind does not do the necessary processing and your body does not recover. This creates both mental and physical health issues. If we are healthy, we can usually cope with the occasional poor night's sleep but it develops into a problem when poor sleep becomes a regular pattern.

When people experience mental health problems, they often lose synchronicity with their normal sleep schedule. Do your best to create a healthy sleep routine.

Things that can upset the circadian rhythm, and therefore sleep, include:

- Travel, especially jet lag
- Anxiety and other mental health problems
- Stress
- Needing the toilet
- Pain
- Physical health problems
- Medication
- Alcohol and drugs
- Eating times
- Shift work
- Noise
- Room temperature, too hot or too cold
- Unstructured bed-time routine (i.e. changing time you go to bed and get up)

Insomnia can also create mental health issues. Only a few weeks ago, my neighbour's dog was barking and barking just as I was trying to get to sleep. My neighbour was out at the time and trying to sort the entire issue raised my stress levels. When I did get to sleep eventually, the quality of the sleep was poor and I kept waking up throughout the night. The next morning, I felt tired, emotional and stressed. If this is the response someone can have to one bad night's sleep, what are the implications of poor-quality sleep for any prolonged period?

Indications suggest adults need between seven and nine hours sleep per night. Few people need more and few can function well on less. This will also depend on our lifestyle. As I have explained, our natural sleep pattern will dip into periods of deeper and then lighter sleep throughout the night. If you cannot achieve the deep sleep, you will most likely feel tired the following day. Some people are naturally light sleepers and it takes very little to disturb them.

If a mental health problem, such as anxiety, means you to struggle to sleep, which in turn causes poor quality rest and recovery, this will exacerbate the mental health issue. I witnessed this recently with one of my clients who had experienced mental health issues for decades but had never addressed them. Eventually he had reached a point when he knew he could not resolve the problem on his own. He contacted me in desperation because he was getting no sleep at all.

Please do not leave it until you reach desperation to seek help because you are suffering for far longer than you need to. It also takes longer to get you back on track.

Sleeping tips

There are many ways to improve your sleep routine. Here are some to try:

- Turn off social media and phone notifications two hours before bed-time.

- Create and adhere to a sleep routine. Sleeping between 10pm and 6am are the best times for recovery.

- Do not eat a large meal within two hours prior to bedtime.

- Some people benefit from a small protein and complex carbohydrate snack about 20 minutes before bedtime. This is because their blood sugar levels drop in the night and this causes them to awaken. For example, an oatcake with nut butter or ham.

- Ensure that your bedroom is at a comfortable temperature.

- Have downtime prior to going to bed. Do not watch adrenalin-inducing television or play computer games.

- Listen to calming music, read a book, meditate or do something relaxing before bedtime.

- Spend a few minutes doing some deep breathing prior to going to bed/sleep.

- Do some exercise during the day.

- Get out in the fresh air, ideally daily.

Stresses of Modern Man

- If you are overweight, start addressing this.

- Avoid caffeine after 3pm.

- Avoid alcohol – make drinking alcohol the exception rather than the rule.

- Change your bedding weekly.

- Some people benefit from a 'grounding' sheet.

- Turn wi-fi off at night.

- Do not take electronic equipment into the bedroom. This can disrupt the energy of sensitive people. If you have been using your phone as an alarm clock, please purchase a specific alarm clock.

- Ensure that the bedroom is suitably dark. Use blackout blinds if necessary.

- Some people benefit from a lavender or magnesium bath prior to bedtime.

- Use protective anti-blue-ray glasses in the two hours before bedtime to aid reduction in cortisol levels.

- Create a healthy work-life balance.

- Address stresses and talk through worries.

- Avoid or cut back on substances such as nicotine, artificial sweeteners, sugar, tea and coffee, fizzy drinks, fried and high fat food.

If you do struggle to sleep here are a few tips which can help:

- Rather than stress about not sleeping, acknowledge that you are getting some rest. Worrying will create stress hormones, whereas if you accept that you are resting, you may find you relax and are able to get back to sleep.

- If noise is a problem, try ear plugs. I find wax ear plugs to be the best.

- Think of something that is blue, such as the sea, an ornament or some other object. Count slowly backwards: "5 – 4 – 3 – 2 – 1 – blue" in your mind. When you get to blue, picture the blue object or scene. Repeat this process. It keeps your mind occupied and bores it into submission.

- Count slowly backwards from 300 to 1. If you lose your place start on the number you remember you were at last or start again at 300.

- Use the tapping technique prior to bedtime with three key words which connect you with sleep such as "sleepy, peaceful, calm". I have included a script in the appendix. When you are in bed you can imagine tapping on the points or tap on the hand points and repeat the words inside your mind. Alternatively say the words without tapping. Repeating them over and over.

- Do some deep breathing. This helps to take you into the parasympathetic nervous system which is the rest and recovery system.

25. Erectile dysfunction

Erectile dysfunction or impotence is more common than you realise. Impotence is the inability to achieve an erection, maintain an erection, or ejaculate consistently. There are both mental and physical reasons for this happening.

The British Association of Urological Surgeons reports that "erectile dysfunction becomes commoner with increasing age and is seen in 50 – 55% of men between 40 and 70 years old".

Possible reasons for erectile dysfunction include:

Medication

Most people do not check the potential side effects when they take their medication for the first time. However, some medications can interfere with blood flow resulting in impotence. Such medications may include those used to treat cancer, heart issues, depression or other conditions. If you experience impotence and believe it may be the result of medication you are taking, speak to your GP so you can discuss the best course of action.

Drugs and alcohol

Any substance abuse could cause impotence, as can over-consumption of alcohol and alcoholism.

Health conditions

Different health conditions linked with the body's ability to pump blood can cause erectile dysfunction. These may include issues related to the heart or diabetes. Diabetes can also cause nerve damage and impact hormone levels.

Information suggests low testosterone levels are rarely a cause of erectile dysfunction, unless there are other relevant health issues. Obesity, high cholesterol and hypertension have also been reported to be problematic. Anatomical abnormalities, such as a tight foreskin, have been reported to be a cause. Trauma or surgery to the pelvic region is occasionally the reason for impotence.

Making the effort to look after your health through limiting stress, exercising and a healthy diet is advisable.

Neurological and nerves

Neurological conditions are diseases of the central and peripheral nervous system. This would be matters of the brain, cranial and peripheral nerves, spinal cord, nerve roots, the autonomic nervous system, neuromuscular junction and muscles. Conditions which fall within this area include diseases such as Alzheimer's and Parkinson's. Other conditions linked with erectile dysfunction include multiple sclerosis, brain or spinal tumours, temporal lobe epilepsy or having a stroke.

Nerve conditions impact the brain's ability to communicate with the reproductive system, resulting in an inability to produce an erection. Nerve damage, including that resulting from prostate surgery, can cause impotence.

Long term pressure on the buttocks and genitals can affect nerve function for men who do a lot of cycling. This can cause impotence, although this may only be temporary. If you cycle and cover a fair mileage, ensure that you are comfortable and do not experience numbness. There are many saddle options and, for the more serious rider, a bike-fit is often beneficial.

Emotional issues

A high number of erectile dysfunction issues are caused by mental health and emotional issues. I would always suggest considering emotional issues as a possible cause first and foremost, unless you know of another obvious reason.

Some common reasons would be:

- **Performance anxiety** – this could be for many reasons. In new relationships, some guys believe their partner is more experienced than they are and are concerned that they will not perform well.

    They sometimes believe they have a partner 'out of their league' or they have 'punched above their weight' and therefore are more self-conscious than usual. This is especially common amongst gay men.

    Any issue where you are concerned about your sexual performance will create anxiety and cause you to over-focus on how you are performing rather than enjoying the moment.

- **Stress** – erections and the processes required to ensure erections happen are all part of our physical system which, just like any other system, requires a healthy hormonal balance, blood flow and a good headspace.

When we are stressed, we are straining one bodily system to fight fire in another bodily system. Something has to give. In this case, it is sexual performance. This stress may be completely unrelated to sex. It could be work-related, family-related or anything else.

- **Depression and the associated fatigue** - can stop you reaching the all-important 'excitement phase' which enables an erection to occur. Also, bear in mind that antidepressants might cause impotence.

- **Anxiety and worries** - can stop you being 'in the moment' or create so much stress around the body that hormonal balance or blood flow do not function properly.

At these times it may be difficult or impossible to achieve an erection when with your partner. You may find that erections will happen sometimes but not always. This can create a cycle of stress and worry around sexual performance, as you then become overly worried about whether you will achieve an erection. This worry will create additional stress and tension.

Despite this stress, you may find that you can have full erections when sleeping and during masturbation.

Options

One option for addressing this is via the medical route, by speaking to your GP. They might ask you a few questions in order to help conclude whether or not this is a stress-related issue. They may also wish to do some tests including blood and urine.

Your GP could also arrange hormonal tests to include testosterone, prolactin, FSH (follicle-stimulating hormone), LH (luteinising hormone) and thyroid hormones.

Through the medical route there are several treatment options. Once your GP has the results, they will then either recommend further tests or a method of treatment.

The other option is to address any underlying emotional issues. Bear in mind that emotional issues may be the underlying cause of any physical problem. The mind and body are undoubtedly connected. One definitely impacts the other.

The root cause might not be related to your relationship or how you feel about your partner, but because of other stresses and problems you face in life. If you are overwhelmed or distracted by problems, this can stop the necessary signals being sent through the body. When under stress, your body increases production of a hormone called epinephrine. Raised levels of epinephrine causes blood vessels to constrict. This interferes with the part of your nervous system responsible for causing an erection.

If you are unaware of any underlying reasons, keep a note of anything which causes you stress over a 10-day period. Also make a note of anything in the past that has happened which might still bother you or may have dented your confidence. These might provide the answers to the underlying cause.

If you seek professional help, a therapist will know to ask you the questions which will uncover anything which may be problematic for you. It makes sense to resolve problems in the most natural way, where possible, through the power of the mind.

This is a personal issue for you but, bear in mind for a therapist, it is about getting to the root of the problem and resolving it. When I see clients for this issue, I treat it just as I do any other issue. More often than not, it is a confidence and performance anxiety issue. It may have started with one night where you struggled to achieve an erection and then became over focused on this memory, causing you to doubt your ability to achieve a future erection.

Here are a few other tips for getting your body in good condition so it is operating at its optimum:

- Remove stress (or reduce as much as possible).
- Resolve emotional issues.
- Spend quality time with your partner, e. g. go for walks or out for meals.
- Be active – exercise four to five times a week. If you have not exercised for a long time, check with your GP to ensure that you are healthy. Increase your exercise routine gradually. Start with brief bursts of exercise every other day and build from there.
- Eat healthily.
- Keep hydrated and drink water.
- Limit alcohol consumption or stop drinking completely for a month.
- Cut back on cigarettes or stop altogether.
- Do some well-being activity such as fishing, pilates, yoga or tai chi.
- Get a massage.
- If you are working long hours, cut back and ensure you have some relaxation time.

The better condition you are in overall in mind, body and emotions, the more likely it is that you will achieve an erection.

26. Anger and aggression

Anger is part of our natural make-up, as are other emotions such as sadness, joy and disgust. Anger becomes a problem when it turns into aggression or when it becomes an emotion you experience frequently. It would be difficult to feel angry and happy or angry and calm. Therefore, if you were to experience anger regularly, it would take away your joy of life. It would be far better to remove yourself from a situation which causes you to feel that way. If that is not possible, then other changes may be possible or perhaps it would help to change your perspective on the situation or develop more positive coping mechanisms.

To be clear on the difference between anger and aggression; anger is an emotion, whilst aggression is the behaviour. This could be a hostile or violent response to a situation or destructive behaviour. Aggression could be verbal threats or insults, which are particularly bad when made in an intimidating manner, such as close to someone's face, towering over them or brandishing a harmful object.

Other aggressive actions could be physical assault, causing damage to property or throwing objects. Some people take the aggression out on themselves through self-harming, which can be quite vicious, such as banging their heads on the ground or a wall for example.

Anger is not always expressed outwardly. We can express anger towards ourselves. As well as self-harming behaviour, this may involve negative self-talk, e.g. telling ourselves we are bad or useless, or self-sabotaging behaviour which stops us being successful or enjoying life to the full.

At the right time aggression can be useful. For example, if someone tried to steal from you, showing aggression may stop that happening and frighten them off. However, aggression becomes a serious problem when it occurs frequently. Perhaps someone has said that you are a very angry person or you know that your reactions are extreme and this is not how you wish to behave.

Anger and aggression have powerful connections to the fight or flight response when stress hormones, adrenalin and cortisol, are released via the adrenal glands.

When angry, most of us do not react physically, for example, by punching someone. Therefore, we do not release those stress hormones. We then spend quite some time stressed about a situation even after the event has occurred. If you are spending a lot of time feeling angry, this could lead to hypertension (high blood pressure) and potentially digestive issues. The emotion needs to be released in a healthy way.

Anger may also be expressed by refusing to speak to someone, ignoring them or being uncooperative. When we take on this type of response it is not aggressive but often leaves us feeling that the issue is unresolved.

In extreme cases, if we take aggression too far, unlawful action could be the outcome. This might be to physically hurt someone, damage their property, or cause harm through a reckless act. The end result could be a prison sentence. Therefore, addressing aggression is vital.

There are many situations which can cause us to feel angry:

- Injustice – is an action of someone right and just in your

opinion? Alternatively, are you being stopped from doing something? This would feel unfair.
- Deceit – someone you trusted let you down.
- Situations you cannot change – traffic jams, government decisions or changes at work.
- Friends and family – behaving in ways you disagree with.
- Personal attack – may be verbal or physical. Also, an attack on friends and family can feel personal.
- Feeling you are not being listened to or understood. You struggle to get your message across.
- Others not acting in accordance with your values. These are extremely important to us. If someone goes against your values, it will create an emotional response. For example, some of my highest values are to act with integrity, to treat people equally and if you say you will do something, then do it.

The above are some examples of what could make you angry. However, the truth is there is no limit to what can make us angry.

Anger becomes a problem when it:

- is aggressive: verbally or physically.
- affects relationships.
- disrupts your family.
- becomes uncontrollable.
- affects your work.
- becomes a frequent occurrence.
- causes others to think of you as an angry person.
- stops you feeling other emotions.
- affects your well-being – mentally or physically.
- takes the joy from life away.

It is important to learn to channel anger in a more balanced way or, when possible, avoid situations which incite anger or aggression.

Sometimes we could relate the anger you feel nowadays to past events in your life. If current circumstances are reminding you of previous situations which were stressful or traumatic, even unconsciously, then this might trigger anger, as an unconscious response.

Aggression may have served you well at some point in life. When a reaction or behaviour such as aggression is helpful in a situation, the subconscious mind makes a note of this. Then, in the future, when you experience a similar situation, your mind will flip to aggression because it recalls that 5 or 10 years ago it was helpful to you. Despite the fact that now the same response might not be the best course of action.

Perhaps aggression was the only way you were successful in defending yourself against an antagonistic parent or a bully. Now, whenever anyone is assertive towards you, which, by the way should be an acceptable behaviour, your subconscious sees this as a threat and kicks into aggression.

Sometimes we need to assess those past events to find a more helpful response that would have served us at the time and going forward. Alternatively, we can accept that the response helped us in that past situation but, going forward, we need a different reaction. We can then consider more appropriate responses to use. In a more relaxed state, we are able to access this information and bring in new perspectives and fresh awareness.

People who express aggression are generally not bad people,

but they have not found more balanced methods to deal with their emotions. They might not feel valued, accepted or have much self-worth.

I have had my own moments of aggression in my life. During my childhood there was a lot of anger and aggression expressed in my family. Over time, it seemed my only available response was anger and aggression, as nothing else worked to resolve the situation. It left me with no other option than to fight fire with fire. However, it was not a positive response or one I liked.

This sometimes became a more immediate response for me when I did not agree with actions and behaviours of others as an adult. I reached a point when I realised that expressing the anger I was feeling in certain situations, albeit verbally, was not serving me. It was creating more conflict and stress for me than I needed or wanted.

I therefore addressed my response through learning techniques such as tai chi and meditation. I started talking through my thoughts and feelings with friends and family. I also became more self-aware. Later, spirituality helped me gain greater understanding of life and brought me more peace. All of this had a calming effect on me, especially because I wanted to feel less anger and stress. I needed another method of dealing with such situations and, with effort, my response changed.

Over time I have also come to accept that many actions in the world are unfair to downright cruel. I am more thoughtful about the battles I wish to fight and use my energy wisely. I decided there was no point getting wound up by all the things I believed were wrong in the world. I can still acknowledge some things are wrong and have empathy and compassion for victims. Save anger for the battles you need to fight and channel it in a way that brings something positive.

Exercise has also been a great stress reliever for me, which can help kick anger and aggression into touch and bring about a more balanced awareness. I find cycling achieves this well for me. An hour or more out in the fresh air with just my thoughts puts me in a kind of trance-like state. In this state, my mind is in a more solution-focused state and often new understandings and ways to deal with situations filter through naturally to my conscious mind.

I recommend outdoor exercise whenever possible. Being out in the fresh air provides an additional level of good feeling. This may be a cycle ride, a walk on the beach, a run or whatever puts you in a pleasant state of mind and gets those stress hormones out of your system. You might find a game of squash or gym session provides that all-important stress relief if you opt for indoors.

Here are some ways to address and manage anger:

- Learn a martial art such as tai chi. Martial arts focus on control and respect. There is a lot to be gained from this type of environment where people are warmly accepted and supported.

- Exercise – a great way to release these stress hormones and gather thoughts. Exercising in the fresh air can be especially beneficial.

- Join a boxing club. This teaches you control and provides a structured outlet for the anger, whilst engaging in a community atmosphere.

- Learn breathing exercises. By creating some mind and body control, you can take charge of your response and generate a more considered reaction.

- Find a good listener with whom you can discuss your frustrations. This may be a therapist, a family member, colleague or friend. Often talking can create a release of tension and the other person may offer some constructive feedback. Sometimes, just to be listened to can be a substantial help.

- Learn assertiveness first – when we act with aggression, the other person is in defensive mode. They are therefore not listening to your words. To be assertive is to address your feelings but to do so by calmly putting your point across. Firstly, consider what outcome you are striving for when you talk to someone. It is useful to say "I feel" so this comes across as less of an attack on the person you are speaking to. Once you have said your piece allow them time to respond. They may have a valid response.

    If they are a reasonable person, they will listen and there follows a productive discussion or perhaps an apology for you. Best-case scenario is that you get your desired response. The worst-case scenario is they are not willing to accept your point of view. If so, walk away and do your best to limit time spent with them in future.

- Begin to recognise your triggers. Sometimes a particular person will easily prompt that anger response, either because you have an unresolved issue with them, i.e. you are still harbouring emotion about something from the past, or they remind you of someone else. Recurring situations might cause anger. Seek to recognise patterns.

- Consider how you can address this. Can you remove yourself from a situation? You might accept that you dislike a certain person or their behaviour but acknowledge this is just the person they are. They may be that way due to events in their past. We are the product of our previous life experiences, including the way we have been treated by others and stressful or traumatic experiences we have had.

- Some people find it helpful to keep a diary of events which trigger anger and aggression. By doing this they can notice patterns and address the underlying issues.

- If drinking alcohol causes you to become angrier and out of control of your emotions, you would be wise to stop altogether or cut back significantly on the amount of alcohol you drink.

- If you are triggered by certain people and it is possible to, try to keep out of their way or spend less time with them. This would be a good strategy.

- Ensure you have a healthy and balanced lifestyle, including food, exercise and relaxation time. This can keep your mind and body more balanced, release stress and help you develop a calmer mentality.

- Meditation helps you develop better self-awareness and gain more control over your mind. You will still have some thoughts during meditation, this is normal. Give yourself time to get used to it. Guided meditations can be great.

- Take 10 deep breaths before responding. This not only calms the body but gives you time to allow the initial flush of emotion to lessen and an opportunity to bring more clarity to your mind.

- Avoid mind-reading. This is when we make assumptions of what others are thinking. It is possible we have it all wrong, so best to ask rather than assume.

- Break the anger state by getting right out of the situation and going for a walk or a bike ride. This can help to move you from the state of anger to understanding what is beneath the emotion.

- Have a 'go to' song which brings you into a positive state such as happiness or calm. You can either play the song in your head or have it available on your phone.

- Connect with a positive image. See the 'calm place' exercise below.

- Use Emotional Freedom Technique (tapping) to release the anger. See the script within the Appendix section.

- Have a simple affirmation that you say when experiencing feelings of anger. For example: "I am at peace and completely calm" or "I breathe out anger, I breathe in calm". You can create your own affirmation too.

Self-reflection

Self-reflection is one of the most useful tools to have in your armoury. Whenever you are triggered by anger, or any other unpleasant feeling or emotion, there are a few questions you could ask yourself in order to bring about more understanding:

- What is it about this situation that bothers me?
- Who does this person/behaviour remind me of?
- What is the repeating pattern in my life?
- Which of my values (an act/behaviour/manner which is important to you) is related to this situation?

Once you have asked yourself any or all of these questions, do not try to force the answer through. It may come straight away or make take a few hours, even days. Every now and then ask the question again, in time the answer should rise to the surface.

This should lead you to understand what you need to let go of and release in order not to be re-triggered. This may take some time if it is strong but be open to change.

Often anger is linked to your past, reminding you of a situation which resulted in unpleasant feelings. Alternatively, it is linked to your values, the things you feel strongly about. When you know the answer, rather than concern yourself with the person or situation that triggered the anger, make it your goal to release the underlying issue in yourself. This can be done through some of the techniques in this book or you may find it beneficial to seek therapy.

If we can bring the trigger back to us then we regain control and can work on our own underlying issues. Whilst the issue is always about someone or something else, then we do not have control and are more likely to be re-triggered. It solves nothing.

Here are a few exercises to help you use your mind more powerfully regarding anger and aggression:

Change your behaviour

Spend a few moments taking yourself into a relaxed state. You can do this by breathing deeply and slowly and, as you do, imagine every part of you relaxing from the top of your head, your neck, shoulders, arms, hands, chest, abdomen, hips, legs down to the tips of your toes. Close your eyes when you are ready.

Picture or imagine a place in your mind where you would feel very relaxed. This might be a real or an imagined place. It could be by the sea, in a meadow or a room with a peaceful ambience. Imagine you are there in the most relaxed state you have ever been in.

Option 1

Once relaxed, recall a time when you were angry or reacted in a way you regret now. Just view this as if you are another person observing yourself. Whether or not you see a clear image, you can connect with the event. You may connect better using your other senses such as feel or hearing.

As you observe yourself, notice how that version of you calms down. They take a few steps back, slow down their breathing and then see how they react differently. Perhaps they walk away or express their feelings calmly. Maybe there is another way you would like them to respond or perhaps they decide not to react at all. What is the new way of responding to the situation? Notice how good that feels for you being in control of your own behaviour.

You have just created an opportunity to change your reaction thereby moving away from anger. To embed this a little deeper, run through that new way of responding another five times. This can be in different situations or run the same scenario through again. This gives your subconscious mind some direction for future behaviour.

Option 2

Once relaxed, recall another time when you were angry or use the same event as for option 1. Now think of someone who you feel would respond in a way which is more helpful. This may be an actor, possibly a film or television character. It may be someone you know personally, such as a family member, colleague or friend.

Now imagine that you take on the personality of that person and respond how you would expect them too. For example, if it were Will Smith, I would imagine he would be relaxed and make light of the situation. If it were Usain Bolt, you can imagine yourself with an enormous smile and moving on, perhaps doing the Lightning Bolt action that Usain did at the end of races. Barack Obama would give a considered yet assertive response. Keanu Reeves would seek to solve the situation by putting others before himself. He would see other people's perspectives. Sir Chris Hoy would stay composed and most likely put some thought into the situation before responding.

Try out other possible responses and consider which works best for you in that situation. Be prepared to try these more positive responses in life situations from now on.

Anger can create an instinctive response of aggression but by using these various measures you can learn to understand yourself and control your response. This way you can take control. Practice really does help embed the new behaviour in your subconscious mind. You can do it.

If sometimes you revert to aggression, do not give up on these practices. Remind yourself that you are in the process of change but not quite there yet. Keep going. In time you will have it under control.

Calm place

Once relaxed, recall a positive memory or create your own relaxing place. This may be a holiday destination, a secret cave you imagine, being in your own garden or anywhere you wish. Mentally take yourself to that place.

Acknowledge what you see all around you. Notice where you are in this place. Are you there alone or are there people or animals with you? What sounds do you hear? Are there any smells? Recognise how you feel to be here. Breathing slowly and deeply through your abdomen. As you are resting in this calming place, take plenty of time to soak up the experience.

Every so often press your thumb and forefinger together to make a connection between that action and these pleasant feelings. Therefore, in the future, when you want to bring back this calmness and connect with your calm place, you find it easier to do so by pressing your thumb and finger together. Take your time to experience this. The more absorbed you are in the experience the better.

Practice equals success

Practice these exercises frequently to make a powerful impression on your subconscious mind. Research suggests it takes 21 repeated efforts for an action to become our natural behaviour. It can also take three times this to break old habits.

27. Depression

Depression can happen to anyone at any time. As with other mental health issues, it does not differentiate between male and female, ethnic origin, financial status, class, sexuality or any other genre.

Depression is known as 'the curse of the strong'. This is because people who suffer depression usually have taken on vast amounts of stress or trauma or are battling through life in some way. They are often the people who help others and put everyone else before themselves. They keep going until something gives and the black cloud of depression descends.

Depression is a message that something is not right and needs to be addressed. When we are not in alignment with our true selves, our health is affected in some way. Unlike sadness, it is not a mood you can pull yourself out of by watching a comedy or going for a walk.

Having depression can cause you to have very low feelings towards yourself. It is not a weakness, but a group of symptoms which happen due to issues which have not been resolved or require healing. People can be deeply depressed yet put on a smile and a brave face for brief periods of time. This means that people they connect with could have no idea what they are going through.

You may fear the response from others if you were to tell them you feel depressed. A response such as "cheer up, it's not that bad" shows a complete lack of understanding of what you are going through. In fairness, why should someone who has no experience of depression understand what it is like and what is needed to recover? However, hearing those words can cause you to feel even worse. It is important that you feel supported and that others acknowledge depression as a genuine illness.

The challenge of most mental illness is that you cannot see it. If you were to break a leg, people could see the cast and offer to help you. They would offer you their seat, hold doors open for you and ask if they can do anything to help. Depression is a hidden illness for many. Some sufferers hide it extremely well.

Thankfully mental health issues are discussed more openly nowadays. This means even if someone does not understand what you are going through, they will realise depression is a real illness and is something which should be addressed.

To guide you further, I will cover the symptoms of depression. Bear in mind that you will, most likely, have some symptoms but not all of them. I have split the list of symptoms between psychological and physical symptoms.

The following list of psychological symptoms appears long because of the underlying issues associated with depression, such as feeling hopeless or helpless. Negative thoughts about yourself are quite common. Remember, you may not have all these symptoms:

Psychological symptoms of depression

- constant low mood or sadness
- feeling hopeless and helpless
- feeling worthless
- poor memory
- lack of patience

- low self-esteem and self-confidence
- feeling tearful
- no desire to socialise
- overcome by feelings of guilt or shame
- feeling irritable
- difficulty concentrating
- intolerant of others
- lack of motivation/everything is a chore
- difficulty making decisions
- feeling agitated
- loss of clarity of thought
- lack of enjoyment in life
- feeling anxious or worried
- negative thoughts about yourself
- negative perception (viewpoint) on life
- thoughts about harming yourself
- suicidal thoughts
- feel isolated or lonely

Physical symptoms of depression

- very low energy
- struggle to sleep/insomnia
- moving more slowly than usual
- decreased (or increased) appetite
- constipation/digestive issues
- low libido
- speech may slow down
- feeling restless
- aches and pains/stiffness

Along with the symptoms are the challenges which a sufferer then faces. Here are some examples of the way your life can then be affected:

Impact on life

- remove yourself from social interaction
- cease participating in hobbies and interests
- relationship difficulties
- addiction/self-medicate
- self-harm
- self-sabotage
- struggle to work
- difficulty getting out of bed in the morning
- eat unhealthily
- weight loss or gain
- stop exercising
- stop looking after your own well-being

Depression can be a lonely place to be if you do not talk to anyone about it. This can cause you to cut off from friends and family, leaving you alone with the negative thoughts as the depressive spiral deepens.

If you believe you might be suffering depression, I do urge you to talk to someone. Sufferers often have such low feelings towards themselves and these need to be put into perspective. Gaining support can help to lift you out of depression.

Depression happens for a reason, even if you do not know that reason. In some way, you took on too much or had to deal with excessive stress or trauma and your limbic system became overloaded. However, through releasing stresses and traumas, using well-being techniques and making lifestyle changes you can rebalance your limbic system and kick depression into touch.

Depression can be a response when feeling hopeless or helpless. People who are in circumstances which they hate, such as a job or family situation, can fall into depression. The solution is to make changes, otherwise you remain in conflict whereby you want to have something different in your life but will not make the changes. This may be because you do not want to upset others, or do not feel in a position to change for some reason. It is possible that you do not feel ready for the change.

As strange as it might sound, I love working with people who suffer depression because addressing the underlying causes really helps sufferers rise out of the darkness. They may always have to look after their well-being and be aware of any triggers for depression to keep on top of it, in the same way that someone who suffers gastro-intestinal issues will do their best to avoid the triggers which upset their digestive system.

What is clinical depression?

Clinical depression is a term used by the medical profession and is considered a more severe form of depression. It references a part of the brain called the limbic system. Our limbic system is critical in our everyday functioning and controls many of the body's processes. The limbic system is also significant in anxiety. It is quite common for those who suffer depression to experience anxiety.

The limbic system also controls our mood. If you put any part of your body under too much stress, it will show signs of strain. The same goes for your limbic system if too much pressure is placed upon it, as the transmitter chemicals tumble under the strain. This then impacts many aspects of day-to-day functioning. These include temperature control, eating patterns, hormonal levels, circadian rhythm (sleep and waking cycle) and mood. This results in suffering any of the symptoms noted earlier.

Clinical depression should not be a life sentence. It should not result in a life-long prescription of antidepressants. I recall talking to one client about their depression as they said "but I am clinically depressed". They believed because of their diagnosis, they could not overcome depression, thinking they could only control it through medication. This is not the case in my experience as a therapist.

Recovery is possible after a clinical diagnosis of depression. The medical profession give illnesses labels to help them and, as society, people are often comforted by labels. In particular, with mental health illness, a diagnosis helps people make sense of what is happening for them.

Medication is not the only option for clinical depression. Far from it. Although occasionally for some, having some antidepressants can serve as a helpful support whilst undergoing therapy and getting back on track. In time, once you are in a better place, it could be possible to gradually reduce the prescription under the guidance of your medical practitioner.

It is possible to kick depression into touch by working through the underlying causes, even if you do not currently know what they are.

What type of people suffer depression?

Depression does not preclude anyone. We are all susceptible

to it. Some may be more susceptible than others. However, there can be a common type of personality who suffer depression. These people tend to be good and caring. Perhaps they care too much about others at the expense of their well-being. Here are a few more personality traits of many sufferers:

- Put others before themselves
- Compassionate and caring
- Concerned what others think of them
- Self-judge
- Take on a lot of responsibility
- Strong morals
- Highly reliable
- Fear judgement from others
- Often 'the strong one'
- Conscientious
- Reliable
- Keep on going no matter what is thrown at them

People who suffer depression are good people but may not appreciate that they should look after themselves better. I know they fear being considered selfish if ever they put themselves first, but I refer to this as self-preservation. It is definitely not selfishness.

Self-preservation is critical
Get yourself in a good place before you help others.

In truth, we cannot look after others if we are not in a good place ourselves. Therefore, it is important to accept that self-preservation is critical. Get yourself in a good place before you sort out other people's problems. It is the right thing to do. In fact, it is the only thing to do.

Seasonal Affective Disorder (SAD)

SAD is a depression which usually surfaces during the autumn and winter months, hence it is sometimes known as 'winter depression'. A few people will suffer with SAD symptoms during the summer and feel better during the winter. However, little is reported about spring and summer SAD.

Women are reported to suffer SAD four times more often than men. However, I wonder if this is purely because men do not report suffering.

There is a connection between the surfacing of SAD and reduced sunlight hours during the shorter autumn and winter days. Lack of sunlight would also result in a reduction in our stored levels of Vitamin D. It is thought that this may contribute to the condition.

The symptoms of SAD are similar to those of depression. The main difference between the two types is that someone who suffers with SAD would feel good during the spring and summer months. This is because there are more daylight hours, more sunshine and we have sufficient Vitamin D. Someone who suffers with depression would continue to experience symptoms throughout the spring and summer months. Sunlight does nothing to lift their mood.

It is reported that this lack of sunlight stops the hypothalamus working properly. The hypothalamus is part of the limbic system and is responsible for the endocrine system. This is a system which includes all the glands in the body, along with the hormones which are produced by those glands. The hypothalamus is also responsible for the nervous system. It is therefore critical in our everyday functioning.

Because of the impact on the hypothalamus, there is a knock-on effect, namely:

Increased production of melatonin – this is a hormone that helps us to feel sleepy. As it begins to get dark, melatonin levels increase. During the winter months, because daylight hours are shorter, some people produce higher levels of melatonin than normal. This causes symptoms of SAD.

Drop in serotonin levels – serotonin is a neurotransmitter which affects mood, appetite and sleep. A lack of sunlight can result in reduced serotonin levels. This leads to the messages not being transmitted through the brain effectively and can result in feelings of depression

Disrupted circadian rhythm – our circadian rhythm is roughly a 24-hour cycle which regulates our sleep cycle, i.e. when we feel sleepy and when we feel awake and alert. It also links with appetite and mood. Less daylight may disrupt the body's natural clock and cause symptoms of depression.

Treatment for SAD

Light therapy – as a SAD sufferer myself, I have found using a lightbox to be incredibly beneficial. If there was only one treatment I was allowed for SAD, I would have my lightbox. The light from these boxes is very bright and is measured in lux. The higher the lux the brighter the light. Lightboxes tend to be in the region of 10,000 lux.

In the depths of winter, I use my lightbox daily. Advice is generally to use for 20-30 minutes a day but I sometimes use for hours and have noticed no adverse effects. Start with 10 minutes and build up to find out what works for you.

I also use a daylight inducing alarm clock, whereby there is a gradual introduction of light in the period before you awaken. This gives your body time to adjust to waking up in the darker months, which makes it less shocking when the alarm goes off. Often the daylight effect wakes me up before the alarm goes off. This is not specifically a treatment, but it is certainly kinder than being awoken to a dark room by a noisy alarm.

Vitamin D – we often talk about topping up our levels of Vitamin D when sat out in the sun or going for a walk in the sunshine. The sun is our best source of Vitamin D. Additionally, some foods provide Vitamin D. These include salmon, herring, tuna, egg yolk, and mushrooms. Some foods are also fortified with Vitamin D. Studies are mixed as to whether Vitamin D is helpful for SAD sufferers. If I notice the effects of SAD kicking in, I will increase my intake of Vitamin D because I believe every little helps.

Holiday – taking a holiday in the sunshine can be a big help for SAD sufferers. After a particularly bad autumn and winter, when it rained nearly every day for 5 months, I suggested to a client who suffers badly with SAD, that he take a holiday in the sun. He did this and when he got back told me that he had felt much better whilst away. The bad news is that once he was back home to a lack of sunlight, it was not long before he was suffering again. I therefore gave him some strict guidelines to follow in using his lightbox more regularly than he had been previously.

Therapy – therapy can help with SAD by dealing with emotions and negative thoughts. One of my clients who suffers badly with SAD responds very well to tapping.

When working with my clients who suffer from SAD, I will always suggest a lightbox and increasing their Vitamin D intake, provided there is no conflict with any medication they are taking. I will also discuss with them other areas where they could make some positive adjustments to well-being such as those mentioned in this book.

Medication – some people will resort to medication for SAD. I believe this should be a last resort, although I never judge people for making a decision to take medication. Selective serotonin reuptake inhibitors (SSRIs) are the preferred type of antidepressant to help treat SAD. These are reported to increase serotonin levels in the brain and improve mood. They will not be effective for everybody and for some, may cause side effects.

Bipolar disorder

Bipolar disorder is a term used to identify dramatic switches in mood and energy between very high and very low. It was once known as manic depression and is sometimes still referred to using this term.

When someone is diagnosed as suffering with bipolar disorder, it can be a defining moment for them in their life. However, I do not believe it needs to be. Bipolar is linked to a layer of the brain called the cortex. There might be other reasons but it can occur when someone experiences frequent or extreme stress or trauma. This may be someone who is sexually, physically or emotionally abused, for example.

There are a few variations in symptoms:

- manic episodes – high energy, thinking and speech

appears erratic (mania is the more severe form that usually lasts for a week or more); or
- hypomanic (a milder version of mania which lasts for a shorter period of a few days usually); and
- depressive episodes (these can be deep lows with severe lack of energy and extremely low mood);
- a sufferer might experience psychotic symptoms during manic or depressed episodes.

There are variations of bipolar, namely bipolar I, bipolar II and cyclothymia which go beyond the scope of this book. Bipolar can impact a sufferer's life in so many ways.

Someone with bipolar disorder may also suffer with anxiety, lack of self-esteem and self-worth. However, they are also amazing people and very capable. It is important to release the negative feelings they have towards themselves, resolve underlying traumas and stresses as long as they are in a suitably balanced state to do so. They also benefit through building in helpful strategies. People who experience bipolar do respond well to holistic treatment. Importantly, they should work with a suitably qualified and experienced professional.

I expect most people who suffer bipolar disorder will have been diagnosed but there are always exceptions. However, my concern is sufferers do not ever have the opportunity to address the underlying issues. If you believe you may suffer from bipolar disorder, then please seek help because it would be immensely difficult to manage without support.

28. Post-traumatic stress disorder

PTSD is the abbreviation for post-traumatic stress disorder. In reality, many people will have experienced PTSD. However, some sufferers will not seek a diagnosis.

PTSD is an anxiety disorder, which can be all-consuming. It occurs after someone is involved in, or witnesses, a traumatic event. Initially recognised in war veterans, now there is no restriction to who might be diagnosed with PTSD. Symptoms can appear years after a period of trauma, e.g. childhood abuse.

Some people are diagnosed with Complex PTSD. This is usually when someone has experienced frequent or regular traumatic events. Someone who has suffered prolonged childhood abuse or been involved in some type of disaster might suffer Complex PTSD.

Often those suffering from PTSD will be in a state of acute anxiety. It is common to experience intrusive thoughts along with any other anxiety symptoms. They are likely to experience flashbacks of the original event. Nightmares or night terrors can occur. It frequently affects sleep, which often causes additional mental and physical health issues.

Being in a constant state of nervous tension will cause the adrenal glands to produce additional stress hormones. This keeps the anxiety symptoms in place and is likely to affect sleep in the long term. Health issues, such as chronic fatigue or fibromyalgia can occur over time.

PTSD may occur years after the traumatic event. This may be due to being triggered by another situation or something which is a subconscious reminder of the initial event. Example triggers can be a person, place, smell, a taste, piece of music or any situation which results in a similar feeling to that experienced when in the traumatic situation.

PTSD may lead to self-sabotaging behaviour. It can also be a catalyst for addictions or other unhealthy coping mechanisms such as OCD or eating disorders. Some people with PTSD cannot hold down a job and they begin to shut off from the world.

Emotions might be extremely mixed. There can be issues of trust and blame apportioned. It is common to experience feelings of shame, guilt or anger. Doing simple tasks, such as going to the shops, becomes a massive undertaking.

Any of your five senses can re-trigger you back into the original event through memory. I recall a story of a war veteran who started to have panic attacks every time he showered. It turns out that the soap his wife had bought had the same scent as the soap he had used during wartime. This took him back to the original trauma, causing the panic attacks.

PTSD can cause irrational behaviour because of the intense stress and fear a sufferer experiences.

Like most mental health issues, there is a reason behind PTSD. Where there is a cause there are solutions. If you suffer PTSD, you may not know it or have not yet been diagnosed with the condition. However, you will be experiencing some unpleasant to damn right awful symptoms. You should not need to suffer. Seek help and support.

29. Obsessive-compulsive disorder

Obsessive-compulsive disorder (OCD) is the diagnosis for someone who experiences obsessive thoughts and compulsive behaviours. A sufferer feels powerless over their thoughts and compulsive actions.

Thoughts and behaviours can vary somewhat between sufferers. Some examples of these would be:

- Flicking a light switch on and off a certain number of times.
- Never stepping on a certain step or stair e.g. the thirteenth.
- Fear over contamination, resulting in extreme cleanliness.
- Intense worry and fear of family members dying or coming to harm.
- Everything must be in order, e.g. tins in the kitchen cupboard, otherwise there may be a thought that something bad will happen.

People with OCD may not trust themselves to have completed some rituals correctly because they have so much self-doubt. This causes them to repeat a ritual many times over. If they cannot be sure they have completed the task correctly, they will start again at the beginning of the ritual. This does frustrate them. However, the underlying fear that something bad will happen if they get it wrong, or need to have control, is too strong to let it go.

In OCD the thoughts are intensely intrusive, as if another force was pushing them onto you, leaving you feeling you have no control over them. They become completely overwhelming for some sufferers. It is not uncommon to believe that your actions can cause a family member to come to harm, be ill or die. Your logical mind may well know this is not the case, but the thoughts are incredibly powerful and dominate any sense of logic.

People who experience OCD may not trust themselves to do everyday tasks such as turn off the oven. They frequently create mantras and behaviours as they complete an action. For example, as you lock the door, you say "everyone is safe" and then spin around three times.

Young children can suffer with types of OCD behaviour. I recall one child who was struggling at school. The teacher kept the child in during break and lunch times to finish their work because they were struggling a little in class. In the child's mind, they were not achieving and may even have considered themselves as bad.

In order that they could achieve, they created a behaviour of collecting items such as sticks and leaves from the garden. This became a daily obsession. They would not rest until they had done so. This was their way of compensating because they were 'failing' in school. However, what the child needed was a feeling of achievement within the school and not to stand out or feel punished for what they found difficult.

This is a good example of how one situation causes someone to develop compulsive behaviour which, on the face of it, appears unhelpful and illogical. However, this was his bid to find a solution, to give him what he needed which was a feeling of achievement. The solution we find is not always logical or helpful and, in terms of OCD, is unlikely to be either of those. However, it is an unconscious process whereby the mind is doing its best to create a solution.

You could say, OCD is a way of creating behaviour which, in a sufferer's mind, keeps them and everyone else safe or is a method of finding some control in life. It can be underpinned by fear. Long-term stress or trauma can be a trigger, as can lack of self-belief. OCD is trying to give you what you are not getting in some other form. This may be safety, comfort, achievement or something else. Therefore, the question is: what is missing or remains unresolved as a situation, period of stress or trauma?

If you are suffering from OCD, be curious what the trigger was for you? I am yet to come across a case where there is no initial trigger.

Some therapies will help you process the thoughts and behaviour consciously and set in motion ways of breaking through these. However, once again, my favoured way of working through OCD has to be through resolution within the subconscious mind. This will, most likely, involve understanding what is behind the disorder and creating the necessary changes. Building up self-esteem, self-worth and confidence are also important, as these tend to be critical factors in OCD.

30. Eating disorders

Men suffering with eating disorders is still rarely spoken about. It is difficult to gain a realistic understanding of statistics given that many men with eating disorders do not seek help.

Common reasons men develop eating disorders include:

- A history of obesity.
- Homosexuality or other gender identification challenges resulting in emotional struggles.
- Involvement in sports which require a lean body type, especially power to weight related or requiring a toned and muscular physique.
- Dieting.
- A relationship breakdown.
- Being bullied or criticised.
- Stresses, e.g. work or studies.
- Family problems, e.g. illness.
- Comments from others about size and shape.
- Lack of self-esteem.
- Media and social media influences.

Nowadays television is frequently centred around appearance. Many guys are ripped (toned and muscular). Body confident men show off their physiques on social media. There is an increasing trend for guys to have a lean and muscular body type. More men are having cosmetic surgery to improve their looks or keep them looking young. The pressure on men to look good has never been so high.

Before the eating disorder starts, often the initial aim is to be healthy, so you may go to the gym and improve your diet.

As you start to enjoy the gains, but want further gains to be quicker, you make more dramatic changes such as increase your exercise and reduce your calorie intake. People notice your weight loss and you enjoy the compliments. There becomes an addictive 'feel good' from the changes, although this is unhealthy and results in the ultimate struggle of an eating disorder.

For men involved in sport, disordered eating can ensue. There is a fine line between disordered eating and an eating disorder. It is so easy to slip from the former, where perhaps you are a little over obsessive, to the latter where the issue has escalated to complete control and strict regimes or you feel out of control of your behaviours.

The main types of eating disorders are:

Anorexia nervosa

Anorexia nervosa is a serious mental illness that results in the person having a very low body weight. This can become life threatening as organs begin to fail. Sufferers have a distorted body image and a powerful fear of gaining weight. They often feel repulsed at the thought of putting weight on, following restrictive diets with minimal calories. They will also embark on exercise routines, although the lack of nourishment and energy will make exercising difficult.

Sufferers often gain great satisfaction from seeing the change in their physical shape. In particular, they gain an unhealthy pleasure in seeing their skeletal structure.

Anorexia is often considered an issue around control. As the sufferer is able to control the food they eat and their weight, they are taking some control over their life. However, other emotional issues can trigger this issue.

If forced to eat, a sufferer may use laxatives to ensure they do not gain weight. Long term use of laxatives can also have health consequences.

Anorexia may be linked to a situation you 'cannot stomach' or 'are unable to digest'. What happened or was said that was very distressing? It can occur after a period of stress and severe lack of self-esteem.

Anorexia is an intense mental health issue. It can be overcome with dedication. The principal obstacle to overcome is a conflict between wanting to be healthy and live a normal life against a strong fear of gaining weight. With the right support, time and dedication you can do it.

Bulimia nervosa

Bulimia nervosa is more commonly diagnosed in males than anorexia. This condition involves bingeing followed by purging. Often the amount of food eaten is excessive. It can result in other health issues and, in serious situations, can become a threat to life.

Sufferers feel as if they have no control over what they eat. They usually go into a trance-like state during the binge and will not recall eating the quantities they have. They certainly do not savour the food.

The purge can occur because of intense feelings of guilt or shame, even disgust towards themselves.

Sufferers will be conscious of their weight and take measures to lose weight including using laxatives, dieting and exercise.

Some people with bulimia will experience periods of normal healthy eating. They may be triggered into a bulimic episode by stress or other emotional issues.

The causes for this disorder are similar to those of anorexia. Overcoming the triggers and boosting self-esteem can help sufferers to achieve a healthy attitude towards food.

Binge eating disorder

Probably more people than we realise suffer with binge eating disorder. Many people binge eat to squash down unwanted emotions. This is, of course, an unhealthy and temporary fix and fails to address the underlying problems.

Bingeing is usually conducted in secret. The desire for food is overwhelming. Often, a sufferer will crave unhealthy food and make a plan to binge, especially if they have an evening in by themselves. Others have told me how they would purchase large bars of chocolate or cake when doing the weekly shop and eat it all on the way home. Due to the shame felt, they would hide the wrappers so their partner, friends or family have no idea how much they have eaten. Just as with bulimia, many sufferers will eat in a trance-like state, often not savouring or even enjoying the food.

Most people who have this disorder will be all too aware of their body size and shape. As they do not purge, they will often put on lots of weight. This adds to the negative feelings they hold towards themselves and because they feel bad, they binge. This is a vicious cycle which becomes difficult to get out of without help.

The same despairing feelings come after a binge such as guilt, misery, shame, regret and disgust.

Reasons for eating disorders

These disorders can be complex and are often linked to other mental health issues. The list of potential reasons for eating disorders are plentiful. Many commence in childhood or teen years. To give you an indication, here are some reasons I have come across through my work:

- As a child, having a strict parent who would not allow you to eat certain foods.
- Being forced to eat food which you hated.
- A traumatic experience (especially around mealtime).
- Being told by a parent that you are too fat.
- Being called 'the chubby one' or some other derogatory term, even if it was meant to be harmless banter.
- Considered that a sibling is more beautiful/handsome than you.
- Not getting attention.
- Sexual abuse or rape.
- Living in a dysfunctional family environment.
- Believing you are underachieving.
- Parents divorcing.
- Bereavement.
- Physical or emotional abuse.
- Suppressed emotions.
- Feeling alone/isolated.
- Lack of self-esteem or self-worth.

Summary

I have known people to flip between eating disorders. For example, someone who was once anorexic may later become bulimic.

If help is sought, it is possible to regain control following a period of binge eating disorder or bulimia fairly quickly, by addressing the underlying issues. That being said, it does come down to each individual's situation. By the time someone addresses anorexia the issues are usually very deeply embedded so may take longer to recover from. It will require commitment on your part. Support from friends and family can be a huge help.

Treatment needs to happen on an individual basis. It is important to understand and heal underlying issues. Dealing with issues around self-worth, confidence and self-esteem are also central to recovery.

This is merely an overview. If you feel you may suffer from an eating disorder, then please seek help. The earlier you can get these issues addressed, the better.

31. Self-harm

People turn to self-harming when they cannot process emotions. This typically involves cutting, scratching or burning, although there can be other actions which cause harm. The act of self-harming causes a temporary release of pressure and can be found to be soothing. For that brief moment, it may silence the thoughts in your head. At the time, self-harming may feel like a soothing switch has been flicked.

Self-harming is not a solution to dealing with pent-up emotions because those emotions keep coming back. This response can be addictive and very difficult to stop. Self-harming can become a coping behaviour for anyone at any point in their life. Although this behaviour will more commonly commence during teenage years or in the early twenties.

Men who self-harm may do so for many reasons, including some of those I have mentioned in this book. The initial causes could be bullying, abuse or a dysfunctional family situation for example, but at the core of it is emotional pain. There may be feelings of hopelessness, shame, guilt, also hatred of self or others.

As a result of self-harming there can come deeper feelings of shame, embarrassment and guilt. These are piled on top of the initial emotions you were trying to quash. It is therefore important to get to the root cause of the emotions and develop healthier coping methods.

There may have been one traumatic event or a series of events which initiated the self-harming behaviour. Your feelings about these can be addressed and released.

It can help to understand your emotions and appreciate that it is okay to feel those. It is fine to feel sad, angry or frustrated. You need not squash these emotions down, but talk to someone so you can find solutions to what is behind those feelings. Sometimes the solution is a chat, alternatively it could be some form of therapy and other times there is a workable solution. Input from others can be invaluable in addressing problems and finding solutions.

There is no definitive list of reasons why someone would self-harm. It can be a response to any situation or emotion. If you are self-harming in the hope someone will notice, this is a cry for help. Please do cry for help and speak to someone. If you find speaking is too difficult, you could send a text, email or some other form of message.

Equally, you may not know the reason behind the self-harming and that is okay too because that can be worked through.

We know that, for many men, talking about their problems and feelings can be a challenge. However, there are a variety of ways that you can address the challenges you are facing in life.

I use some 'contentless' therapies. This means you need not tell me what the event is which comes to mind or the situations you are struggling with. Therefore, if you are humiliated, embarrassed or feel guilty about an event from your past and this is stopping you from seeking help, you need to know that there are methods available to address it without you telling a therapist what it is. I have noted types of therapies, which can be used in a contentless format, under the FAQ section.

A good therapist will listen and make the effort to understand you. Plenty of holistic therapies are not in the game of analysing or categorising you, but are available to create the changes you need in a supportive manner. Keep an open mind because you might be surprised at what is possible.

32. Suicidal thoughts

Some people would prefer not to be in this world any longer and have thoughts about ending their life. Perhaps more people than we realise. Those thoughts may be nothing more than a fleeting moment. It is a small number of people who carry those thoughts further into considering committing suicide and how they will go about it.

Some talk about people attempting suicide as a call for help. This can be the case. Others may make an attempt to end their life and then regret it instantly. They will then call someone and tell them what they have done. For others, the attempt will be successful.

If you experience suicidal thoughts and believe that you may carry those thoughts through, then it is imperative that you seek help immediately. I have included some contact details in the Appendix.

When you do talk to someone, they will not have all the answers straight away. However, if they can sit with you or be on the phone with you then progress can be made. You know you have their support. From there, further help and guidance can be gathered.

You could complete the communication form in the Appendix section and share this with someone prior to talking. Alternatively, pass it to them when you speak.

Bear in mind, if you are taking medication it is possible that this is contributing to the way you feel, especially if you are taking more than one medication. Therefore, please speak to your GP or consultant to be sure this is not the case as a simple fix might be possible.

Having thoughts about suicide usually comes after a period of struggling with a build-up of emotions or following a dramatic event in your life which, at the time, you believe you cannot move on from. Sometimes you believe you are in a situation you cannot get out of. This can cause feelings of helplessness and hopelessness, but time does not stand still and change is possible.

For some, the suicidal thoughts seem uncontrollable. It is as if there is a voice in your head, which is separate to you, saying negative things such as:

- You are worthless.
- Nobody loves you.
- You're a bad person.
- You must end it all now.

However, these are all false. The truth is:

- You are worthy.
- People do love you.
- You are a good person.
- There is much to live for.

Sometimes people feel suicidal because the intense negative thoughts they have are so overpowering they feel they can no longer live with them.

It is important to understand that whatever those negative thoughts are; they are a misconception; they are an incorrect perspective of you and your life. These thoughts might be comments made by other people based on their misguided ideas. They could be your own thoughts because you have lost perspective on how amazing you are and what is truly possible.

The truth is:

- People do love you.
- People would miss you if you were not here.
- Others would have wanted you to tell them how you are feeling so they could help, even people you are not close to.
- There is so much to live for.
- Others have felt as you do but have come out the other end and now have a good life. They are grateful that they did not end their life. They just needed to know that the way they felt would not be forever. Please know that it won't be forever.
- People are not bad, sometimes they do bad things but they can make up for their actions.
- You can change the direction of your life at any time.
- You are worthy and capable. You have a bright future if you allow yourself this opportunity to turn the corner.
- The way you feel right now is not the way you will feel forever.
- This is the darkest moment. However, on the other side of this is a much brighter life.

Suicidal thoughts are not permanent but at the time they feel all-consuming. They suggest there is no alternative but the truth is, there is another possibility. There is always another option. When you exit the dark tunnel, there is light. Suicidal thoughts are the dark tunnel, keep moving through. Every tunnel has an exit.

The better option is to live and change what is causing you this pain. This may be to change a situation you are in, or to release negativity you are holding due to life experiences or for other reasons. You will need some guidance to do this. The first step is to accept that change is possible. It truly is possible.

Most people who feel suicidal will be able to move on given time and help. They go on to live contented and fulfilled lives.

Those suicidal thoughts are like a deep cut in your mind but even the deepest cut can heal given time and support.

Other people may not be aware that you are feeling suicidal. Please do not assume they will know how you are feeling but do not care. Often when people have suicidal thoughts, they are able to cover them up and even appear happy to others. In fact, many people appear happy just before they commit suicide because they have made a decision to end it all. This gives them closure and, with closure, comes peace of mind.

Dark night of the soul

We have a bottle in our Colour Mirrors system called Illumination. Through the Colours Mirrors I have been able to experience life in a new way. The system has guided me to let go of patterns that do not serve me. It helps to bring a fresh perspective on experiences. In brief, the system is about releasing everything which does not serve us and bringing in peace, love, joy and many other good vibes.

I want to share this with you through the G8 Illumination bottle. This is about having the faith to know that the darkness you are currently experiencing is part of your life experience but you know you will move beyond it out of the dark and back into the light. In the light you will be able to use your learnings and experiences in a positive way.

Consider now what that light will look like and the life you will then create. What appear to be obstacles currently are the negative beliefs you hold. They are where your focus is but they are not the truth. Imagine if you could step over everything holding you in this place, or if you were to release those negative beliefs and create a more joyful and peaceful reality. This is truly possible. People before you have done so, therefore, so can you.

Exercise

Spend a few moments considering this brighter future. Consider the questions below then close your eyes and start to imagine the life you want:

- What would a brighter future look like for you? What do you see?
- What sounds do you hear?
- What would that future feel like?
- How do you want to experience your future?

Now consider the first step to making this brighter future.

Set yourself a plan to start creating this more positive future.

- Consider what you are passionate about.
- What do you enjoy spending your time doing?
- What brings peace in your heart and mind?

It is time to start creating the life you want. Take back the power, then begin the first steps towards the future you desire. Every success story starts with one small change. Take your time with the above exercise. Go over it in the days ahead and expand on it. If you are creative, use those skills. If you are a checklist type of person then write out a checklist and start taking action.

Here is the wording for the Illumination bottle:

> "This bottle is the darkest of the entire range. It supports you as you go into the heart of darkness in your subconscious and begin to feel the warmth and depth of the love that exists there. This is the seat of all potential. It is the moment when sleep finally overtakes you. The void. The place of dreams. This bottle is called Illumination, as it is only by going into the darkness and embracing it that you have the potential to step into the light. As you accept your shadow, you release your fears and judgements about the unspeakable that you hold within.
>
> This bottle brings to light the unhelpful beliefs and judgements you have been holding about your physical body and supports you in transforming them. It helps clear your genetic line of the physical, emotional and karmic patterns you have inherited. The 'sins' of the fathers can no longer be visited on the children once the past darkness has been illuminated. As you face your shadow, you can move beyond it to a place where you create a reality based on the light rather than the dark. Everything you have in your life exists because you created it, albeit unconsciously. Now is the time to become a conscious creator and focus on what you truly wish to create – and this bottle is the ultimate support. Let it help you clear unconscious blocks and return to clarity so that you can claim your absolute magnificence."

Section 3
Creating good mental health

Now you have the background, you can start to make changes.

You have the knowledge.

Now take action to create the best life possible.

33. The road to recovery

One thing is for sure. To feel better, something needs to change. You will need to take some action. This may be to seek therapeutic support, change your lifestyle, remove yourself from negative people, include well-being activities in your day or something else entirely. You probably have a good idea what needs to change. However, you might not know how to feel better yet but, through the course of this book, you will have gained some useful insights.

This next section is to give you information and support. I suggest you attempt all exercises. You will find greater success with some more than others. In which case, continue with those exercises. Although we want instant success, getting better is rarely a quick fix. However, it is a worthwhile journey and commitment does pay off. Invest in yourself. You deserve it.

Sometimes you make a change or do a well-being exercise and feel 2% or 5% better. If you continue with the exercises over a period of time, these percentages add up. There can come a point when you think "I feel great". Sometimes when we feel really bad, it is hard to believe we can turn the corner, but it is possible.

Whatever condition someone is in when they first come to see me, I keep an open mind as to what is possible. They might ask me how many sessions they will need. I can never give them a precise number because I need to see how they respond to the work we do and gain a greater insight into what needs to be resolved. There are times when I am amazed at the speed of improvement from someone. This can be due to working on one key event. We release the stress or trauma and the response is powerful.

Just as with physical health conditions, once you feel better, you may need a 'maintenance' programme to ensure that you stay in good mental health. Maintenance usually requires less time out of your day or week than the initial healing phase. Once you are in that good place you will have completed the bulk of work but do not become complacent. Going forward, you may find that 10 minutes of focused well-being a day or a couple of helpful activities a week keeps you in a good place.

The first area to slip when we are busy is looking after ourselves. Yet this is the most important thing we can do. Continue to check in with yourself and how you are feeling and be aware of the signs which are telling you things are slipping. It is far easier to address problems and difficulties at an early stage. That way you can be back to feeling good much quicker.

What you focus on is important. Please believe that you can achieve good mental health. Think about the life you want and how you will get there. Right now, you might not have all the tools to get yourself there but keep learning and seek support where needed.

Invest in your own recovery. Be patient with results.

Always look after all aspects of your health.

34. General well-being

General well-being is essential to good mental health. If we are physically unwell, it affects our mental health and vice versa. So, let's start with the basics.

Eat healthily

Most people understand, even on a basic level, what food is good for them and what is less healthy. Here are some very simple tips to ensure that you are supporting your well-being through a sensible diet:

- Eat three main meals a day - breakfast, lunch and dinner.
- Ensure you include a variety of colourful fruit and vegetables in your diet.
- Limit sugar intake. Sugar is in many processed foods.
- Eat wholegrain foods.
- Consume food in its natural state, rather than processed, most of the time.
- Limit fizzy drinks to a maximum of one a day.
- Do not drink caffeine after 3 pm.
- Do not eat a large meal two hours before bedtime.
- Eat protein with every meal.
- Drink water and keep hydrated.

When working with my clients on healthy eating, I never seek 'perfection'. If you eat a little processed food, then it is unlikely to cause you any harm. There are a lot of people who miss breakfast. This can cause weight gain and play havoc with metabolism. Skipping meals usually results in eating more food later on in the day when you are less likely to burn it off. It can also result in fatigue and lack of concentration.

Water is of significant benefit to health, so I encourage you to drink it. If you are not a fan of plain water, try it hot or warm. It is surprisingly palatable.

Recommendations are to drink approximately two litres of water a day. However, this does depend on many factors including your size, how much you perspire and lose in other ways. Two litres is a good starting point. If you are firm in not wanting to drink water on its own then add some cordial or try herbal teas. Hydration is very important.

If the above all seems too challenging right now, make small adjustments to your lifestyle each day.

Food intolerance

Sometimes we become intolerant to certain foods. This may be a lifelong intolerance or for just a few months. When we are stressed, it is more likely that our body links some foods to stress and sees them as invaders.

If we suffer with food intolerance, this can cause us to feel lethargic, impact the gastrointestinal tract and therefore digestion and bowel movements, upset our mood, creating anxiety and cause other unpleasant responses. It can be worth investing in a food intolerance test. The most accurate test is a blood-related test. Other types of tests can be less reliable.

The blood test is usually conducted as a home kit, whereby you create a minor cut in a finger and use the swab provided to take the blood sample. You then send the sample to the laboratory. Usually within approximately 7-10 days you will receive information regarding any intolerances.

By eliminating foods which you are intolerant to, you may find an improvement both physically and mentally, as I did. You may not need to rule these foods out of your diet forever. Sometimes avoiding them for a number of months can help your body to reset.

Please note that intolerance is different to an allergy. An allergy creates a rapid response from the immune system. You will have a quick, and often dramatic, reaction to certain foods. This may be within seconds or minutes of exposure to the allergen. The most common of these are nuts, shellfish, dairy, wheat (gluten) and strawberries.

Response to food intolerance is usually more subtle although, if not addressed over time, can become problematic especially if the range of foods you become intolerant to increases.

Another way to assess food intolerance is through an elimination diet. This is where you would omit certain foods and food groups.

After eliminating those foods for a period of time, you reintroduce them very slowly and in small amounts to give you an opportunity to notice whether there is any reaction. The recommended elimination period can vary but is often six months to enable your physical system to recover and reset.

There are different methods for elimination diets. You may wish to consult with a nutritional therapist on this. Alternatively, there is plenty of literature available.

It can be easy to cast this idea aside but I can talk through my own experience. I was at a point of feeling dreadful. My digestion was awful, I was constantly exhausted, my heart was racing and my body was tingling. I heard about food intolerance testing so I took the plunge and had a test. The results were astounding. I was intolerant to a huge number of foods. There were so many problem foods for me that I could not wipe them all out of my diet. However, I removed about 95% of those flagged, found replacements and within 10 days felt noticeably better.

My results were extreme. This was during a long period of burn out. The intolerance was one way my body was reacting to burn out, and trying to tell me to stop. It did not resolve all the burn-out symptoms, as I had to make further lifestyle adjustments, but it certainly helped to improve my well-being. Now, I can say happily that many foods have been reintroduced to my diet albeit carefully. Some of which I never expected I would eat again.

I have not taken a test for some time but monitor how I feel and am conscious to eat specific foods in only very small quantities. I also know the main culprits from my previous results and how I react to some foods. If I were to start to feel bad or notice reactions, I could make a decision to cut certain foods out and may not have a need to re-test.

If you suspect that food intolerance might be an issue for you then it can be worth proceeding with a test or elimination diet. It is worth the effort.

Exercise

When it comes to well-being, exercise is essential. It helps us mentally and physically. Through exercise we release stress and raise our mood.

Exercising can involve going out in the fresh air, which can make us feel good. Even on a chilly day, as long as we have appropriate attire, getting outside for anything from 20 minutes to a number of hours helps us to feel good.

During exercise neurotransmitters, known as endorphins, are released, causing a positive change in the brain chemistry. Endorphins are reported to be structurally similar to morphine and can therefore provide pain relief and feelings of well-being. Therefore, after exercising, many people report that they experience a more positive mood and sense of well-being. This is certainly the case for me. Exercise helps me feel as if I can deal with whatever the day brings. Regular exercise is also reported to create a greater feeling of self-control and raise self-esteem.

When you exercise, it does not have to involve building up a sweat and getting completely out of breath if you prefer not to. You are no longer in the school playground being shouted at by your physical education teacher. Therefore, you get to choose what exercise you include in your wellness plan.

I know some men have found it beneficial to join groups or teams. You may also form good friendships in these groups and find a confidante who you are at ease chatting too.

When I go out riding on my bicycle, I am sorting through all my thoughts and any concerns I have, I am also at my most creative. This is because I am in a more relaxed state of mind. When I get home, I feel much lighter in my mind and mood. If, for any reason, I cannot exercise for a few days, I notice that I am less chirpy and my mind is more cluttered. There are definite mindset benefits to exercising.

Do activities you enjoy and connect with. If you hate the gym, then do not go. If exercise has never been your thing, then explore the many possibilities. I promise when you find something you enjoy it is fun. You may well surprise yourself.

If you are unfit and have not exercised for some time, you may wish to have a check-up with your GP. I always advise to start gently and build up as you get fitter. This may be a 10-minute walk around the block at first. If you are unfit, and especially if you are overweight, it is important that you do take your time to build your fitness to ensure you steer clear of injury. You are also more likely to continue with exercise if you incorporate it into your lifestyle rather than have a get fit quick attitude.

Grounding

The term 'grounding' (or 'earthing') has become such a well-used term. I am concerned that people ignore its importance to our mental and physical health and well-being. In particular, grounding has been beneficial for those who suffer anxiety. Again, if we go back to our ancestry, we did not wear shoes so grounding was something we did naturally and took for granted. We are victims of our own evolution now that we wear shoes which prevent us from grounding naturally.

To a great extent the stress and anxiety people experience results from a disconnection between mind, body and earth. By being better connected in these areas, you will experience a greater sense of well-being.

People sometimes think of grounding as something hippies do, but it has health benefits. There is scientific backing to its benefits.

The interchangeable terms earthing and grounding refer to the act of walking barefoot on the earth. This allows the transfer of free electrons from the earth into your body, through the soles of your feet.

When we are disconnected from the earth, our bodies do not hold a negative charge effectively. Our brains are also less effective and therefore the communication between mind and body becomes compromised. Our brains function much better when our electrical systems work better.

Signs of being ungrounded

Mental signs:

- Anxious
- Over-thinking
- Constant worrying
- Feeling spaced out or absent-minded
- Easily distracted
- Over-dramatic

Physical signs:

- Poor sleep/insomnia
- Inflammation
- Chronic pain
- Fatigue
- Poor circulation

Grounding can help to reverse the damage caused by electro-magnetic fields (EMFs) and other types of radiation from Wi-Fi, mobile phones, computers and other damaging technology.

Another benefit is that grounding reduces inflammation. When our bodies are positively charged, the blood is thick and the cells of our bodies are trying to battle against free radicals. Grounding puts the body in its preferred state of being, which is slightly negatively charged. This alleviates inflammation as the blood becomes thinner. Grounding is a key component in the foundation of good health and well-being.

I used to have a very unsettling feeling through my body. The best way to describe it was like an electrical current going through parts of my body, especially my limbs. Once I started to ground myself, this disappeared and I had a greater sense of well-being.

There are many reported benefits to grounding, which include:

- Reduces emotional stress
- Elevates mood
- Improves sleep
- Increases energy
- Helps support adrenal health function
- Improves sense of wellness
- Reduces inflammation
- Reduces chronic pain
- Relieves muscle tension and headaches
- Aids and often speeds up healing
- Reduces jet lag symptoms
- Protects the body from the effects of EMFs
- Decreases recovery time from injury
- Reduces snoring
- Normalises biological rhythms
- Normalises blood pressure and blood flow

There are different methods for grounding. I encourage you to try these out.

Barefoot walking

Our ancestors used to walk around barefoot, which means they were always grounded. This suggests being ungrounded is a symptom of modern living. By grounding through direct contact with the earth, we can reinstate our body to its natural state of a slight negative charge. Barefoot walking helps us to absorb the nutrients of the earth. The very best place to do this is to walk on the beach and paddle your feet in the water, which is a great conductor of energy.

Another method for grounding is to walk on grass. When walking barefoot, please be careful to ensure you are walking in a safe place away from anything and anywhere that could cause injury.

Bathing

Nothing beats a swim in the sea for grounding and the impact on your well-being. Alternatively, bathing or using a foot spa containing Epsom salts and/or Himalayan salts is a lovely relaxing way to ground yourself.

Grounding mat or sheet

A grounding (or earthing) mat can be used under your feet while using a computer, which reduces your vulnerability to the EMFs. Many grounding mats come with a wrist strap option.

Note: when using grounding mats while working on computers, if your computer is plugged in, you may create a positive charge. To avoid this, ensure your computer is not plugged in, therefore only ground yourself when the computer is working in battery mode. In my experience, MacBooks are best unplugged when working on them in any event.

My preference is a grounding bed sheet because I have found greater benefit to this than the grounding mat. A sheet provides a fantastic eight hours of grounding while sleeping. To gain the greatest benefit, you would need to be naked, or mostly naked, so your skin is in contact with the sheet. It is worth buying a quality grounding sheet.

Start by creating a basic, balanced lifestyle.

Create time for you because you are important.

35. Well-being activities

Life is busy, which means we have to take the time and effort to incorporate well-being activities into our day. Essentially activity has an impact on our energy levels. It either drains us or rejuvenates us.

In most cases well-being activity is connected to the parasympathetic nervous system, in order that you achieve recovery and healing. I say 'most cases' because occasionally to incorporate something filled with adrenalin can be good if it lifts your mood. However, too much adrenalin-filled activity will drain your physical and mental health. Therefore, this type of activity should be limited. For this reason, I am focusing more on relaxing activities because these will enhance your health.

You should enjoy your well-being activities. They should not be a chore. However, initially, they may appear strange and you might think you are wasting your time because you could do more 'beneficial' things such as working or some DIY. However, please do not under-estimate the benefit of taking well-being seriously and making it a part of your life.

One activity I do for my well-being is making beaded jewellery. I can get lost in it for an hour or more. When I am making the jewellery, my mind is zoned out from everything else. It is quiet from thoughts and focused solely on the activity, which is a healthy state to be in.

One of my clients does jigsaw puzzles. At first, he found it a challenge to allow himself that time to relax into something he considered unproductive. However, he soon found it an enjoyable experience and appreciated the benefits to his well-being. By becoming absorbed in the pastime, it cleared his mind of thoughts in the process. Doing an activity similar to this is a detox for the mind. You are allowing the brain some downtime. This is vitally important for good mental and emotional health.

We need to move away from our programmed thoughts about how we use our time. There is no better use of your time than to look after your well-being. We do not need to always be earning money or doing something productive. Sometimes we need to sit back, calm the mind and breathe.

We have become so used to being prescribed medication. We convince ourselves this is fixing us but at best the medication hides the symptoms and at worst it makes you feel even more dreadful than you did without it.

We are not powerless to improve our health and well-being. Therefore, we can take positive action. This does require us to be proactive and to commit to helping ourselves. It is empowering to create your own solutions and become more in tune with yourself.

Often when we become sick, we cannot recognise the cause or what makes us feel good because we become so jumbled up. However, as healing takes place, we are more able to recognise what causes us to feel bad. We can also notice what makes us feel good. This helps us to become more proactive and make important decisions to take better care of our own health.

For these reasons, I am listing below some well-being activities you might like to try. Of course, if you have other ideas then please do try them out.

- Singing
- A soak in the bath
- Cuddling up to your pets
- Listen to some soothing music
- Do a jigsaw puzzle
- Model making
- Tinker with a vehicle
- Paint or draw
- Play a musical instrument
- Walk
- Swim
- Spa treatments/massage
- Sauna or jacuzzi
- Colouring
- Cooking/baking
- Gardening
- Writing e.g. music, poems
- Reading
- Meditation
- Yoga
- Bicycle or motorbike ride
- Listening to an audio book/podcast
- Socialising with friends
- Art gallery/museum

The principle of well-being activities is that they should soothe you. They should take your mind out of the negative thoughts and worries. If you are not used to doing anything like this, it might seem strange for the first few occasions. You may think you should do something 'more productive' but please persevere because it is important and could just be the most significant thing you do all week. Over time you will appreciate the benefits of taking this time for you and prioritise well-being activities.

Empower yourself to improve your mental, emotional and physical health through well-being activities.

36. Power of the breath

We breathe every day, many times a day. However, we do not always breathe in the healthiest way, especially when under stress. Daily living with its associated stress and worries has caused people to lose touch with their natural way of breathing.

Most of us will be using just a tiny portion of our lungs to breathe. Through our challenging and busy lifestyles, we become tense. Our breathing rate increases as the depth of breath lessens. Quality breathing will put you into a more parasympathetic (relaxed) state, creating good mental and physical health.

It helps to incorporate focused breathing into your daily routine.

Deep abdominal breathing

The technique:

Step 1

You may find standing is the best way to do this exercise until it comes easily. This breathing method is all done through the nose, unless you have any nasal issues, in which case you can breathe through your mouth.

Place one hand on your chest and one hand on your abdomen. When you breathe using your entire lung capacity, your chest hardly moves as your abdomen expands on the in breath. Therefore, the hand on your chest should hardly move, but the one on your abdomen should move quite noticeably as you breathe in.

Close your mouth and imagine that you are blowing up a balloon in your belly. As you take a slow and steady, deep breath in through your nose, your abdomen should expand because the air is going in. When you breathe out the air goes out of your abdomen and therefore it deflates. To recap, your abdomen expands on the in breath, like a balloon, and deflates on the out breath. Breathe in for the count of 5 and out for the count of 5.

If you are struggling to connect with the deep breaths, do a very brief powerful breath into your belly so you can connect with that area and then you will be able to do the slower breaths. Do not worry if it takes you a while before you get the hang of it. Please persevere.

Step 2

Now slow the breaths down. The aim is to breathe in for the count of seven and out for the count of eleven. Repeat those slow and deep breaths as they will calm your nervous system down.

How to use the deep breathing

Here are a few options for using deep breathing. Ensure you do some every day.

1. Spend five minutes focusing on deep breathing at a slow and steady pace.
2. After you complete a task, do two slow and deep breaths. For example, when you make a drink do two of these

breaths, when you go to the toilet do two of these breaths and so on.
3. When you are stuck in traffic, in a queue or sat waiting for an appointment do some deep breathing.
4. When you worry or feel anxious, take deep breaths. When you make deep breathing part of your daily practice, doing so in times of worry or anxiety will be easier because you will be well-practiced.

Through focused breathing, we can come back to the moment we are in and remind ourselves that all is well.

Breathing exercises

Select one of these for your daily breathing exercises. Feel free to inter-change between these if you like variety. You can carry out these exercises lying down, sitting or standing.

4-7-8 relaxing breath

The 4-7-8 breathing technique, also known as "relaxing breath". Here is how it works:

Rest your tongue on the bottom of your mouth during the exercise. This helps to relax your jaw muscles. To start with exhale completely through your mouth.

- Close your mouth and inhale through your nose for a count of four.
- Hold your breath for a count of seven.
- Exhale completely through your mouth for a count of eight.

Do this for 2 - 5 minutes.

Equal breathing

Quite simply, make your inhales and exhales the same length. Once again, breathe deeply, using your lungs more completely.

If you have a small set of lungs, you may prefer to do this to the count of four. Someone with a larger set of lungs may be comfortable counting to six. This should feel pleasant and calming.

- Breathe in and out through your nose.
- Count to four (or whatever number you decide) as you inhale.
- Pause for a brief moment (one or two seconds)
- Count to four (or whatever number you decide) as you exhale.

As you become more accustomed to this type of breathing, you may prefer not to count but to focus on those steady and even breaths. This can be incredibly relaxing.

Do this for 2 - 5 minutes.

Whole body breathing

Once again this is deep and slow breathing. As you take a breath in, notice how your lungs fill and your upper body lifts slightly. Imagine your entire body benefitting from this healing breath.

As you breathe out your upper body relaxes and, as it does, tension releases too. Imagine all tension in your body and mind releasing.

You may like to use the word "calm" on the inhale and "release" on the exhale by repeating this to yourself inside your mind.

Do this for 2 - 5 minutes.

Summary

Deep breathing is a great way to start and finish the day. Some focused deep breathing in the middle of the day can help to reset the equilibrium. If you struggle to sleep at night, do some deep breathing. Never underestimate the importance of this. It helps to calm down your nervous system and brings in better clarity of thought.

Practice deep breathing every day.

It's very important.

37. Affirm the positive

What we tell ourselves is important. When people experience mental health problems, they focus on the negative and have internal conversations which are pessimistic, even destructive.

You might tell yourself you are a bad person or you will have a crap day, or repeat that you are useless or a waste of space. Of course, this will make you feel bad. It is a form of self-sabotaging behaviour, even when unintentional.

It is important that what you tell yourself is positive, supportive and encouraging, with a view to creating the life you want for yourself. We will look at positive self-talk using affirmations.

Personal affirmation

I understand that being positive towards yourself can be challenging, especially if you hold a belief system which is telling you the opposite. You do not have to believe the affirmations in order to introduce them into your self-talk. Here are some examples:

- I am a capable person
- I believe in myself
- I am likeable
- I am a good person
- I am successful

Consider what you want to bring into your life. You can use any of my suggestions above or create an affirmation of your own.

Once you have decided on your affirmation, say this either out loud or inside your mind every day, three times when you wake up in the morning and at night before you go to sleep. Say the affirmation as if it is absolutely true, regardless of what you believe. Additionally, repeat the affirmation to yourself periodically throughout the day.

You could look at it this way. We all have inner self-talk. Those ramblings going on in our mind throughout the day. We can talk to ourselves in a negative and unhelpful way, which brings us down, or we can talk to ourselves in a positive and helpful way, which lifts us up. In terms of mental health, it is vitally important to do the latter.

Life affirmation

When we are unhealthy in mind or body, we tend to place our awareness on the negativities of our situation and how bad we feel. This just reinforces everything we do not want.

An affirmation is an excellent way to help us focus more positively. It also helps to direct our attention, and therefore energy, on what we do want in life. This simple action is giving your mind helpful guidance. Here are some options:

- I feel good every day
- Life is positive
- I am getting better each day
- I choose to live a happy and joyous life
- I seek the positive in every situation
- Life is full of opportunities.

Use your life affirmation every day. You might use it when you first wake up or when you are waiting, such as on the toilet, in a queue, driving or waiting for an appointment. Feel free to create your own personalised affirmation.

Situation affirmation

There could be a specific event coming up or a situation you are going through where you will benefit from creating a specific affirmation, perhaps for a short period of time. This might be related to a job you have applied for, an event you are taking part in, a person, or something else entirely.

Here are a few examples:

- I have the skills for this job.
- I am fit and ready to run 5 km.
- People are going to love my speech.
- I am calm when in the company of my in-laws.
- I am ready for this promotion and going to show them just how capable I am.

Summary

The more positivity you can create in your mind the better. If you do not believe the affirmation, be open to it happening for you. When you do say it, either out loud or inside your mind, do so with commitment. Say it in a way that makes it the absolute truth. Your subconscious is always listening, therefore give it something positive to listen to.

Repetition is a way of forming new beliefs so keep doing it. It is important for you to encourage yourself towards feeling good. Every time you speak to yourself in an encouraging, supportive and positive manner, you are paving the way for a better life.

Speak to yourself in an encouraging, supportive and positive manner by creating daily affirmations.

38. Seek out the positive

Gratitude is great for creating a more positive state of mind. In terms of our physical condition, it can also help for healthy information to flow through the cells of our bodies, putting us in a wholesome state. A thought carries an energy which our body tunes into. Hence creating positively-focused thoughts is important for good health in mind and body.

During the coronavirus (Covid-19) outbreak in 2020, many individuals focussed on the positives and the good things they had in their lives. They made the most of the enforced changes. Other people would draw attention to what they were not allowed to do or the things they did not have.

Many people shared bad news and negativity with no consideration for how it might affect others. This created fear, frustration and much negativity in society.

My view on what I shared was it had to be true, positive or helpful. If it was none of those then it was important for me to consider why I would share it. The same goes for your well-being. A flow of positive information from both yourself and external sources is most beneficial, even when times are difficult. This means that finding the positive in any situation is going to create a healthier mindset than focusing on the negative.

It is beneficial to consider things you are grateful for on a frequent basis. Even if you have little in your life, there are still many things you can be grateful for.

"Wherever you go, no matter what the weather, always bring your own sunshine."

Anthony J. D'Angelo
Author & Founder of Collegiate EmPowerment

Another good use of your mind is when you notice someone else talking in a negative manner, create a positive response. This encourages your brain to work in a more optimistic and upbeat way. By these actions, you are getting the best use of your mind and training your brain to work for you rather than against you.

As part of your well-being plan, I would like you to think of three things you are grateful for daily. It does not matter if you express appreciation for the same things two days in a row, the important thing here is the connection to gratitude and the good vibes it creates.

There is no restriction or limit on what you can be grateful for. Today I am grateful for the sunshine, spending time with my cats and an enjoyable cycle ride I had. You could be grateful for a nice coffee you had, a TV programme which entertains you or a jacket you like. The options for gratitude are endless. You do not need to wait for the big lottery win to be grateful. Gratitude for the small things in life is priceless.

To make a start, for the next seven days at the end of each day make a note of three things you are grateful for. Aim to make this part of your daily routine ideally continuing past those seven days.

Practice gratitude daily and seek out the positives in all situations.

39. Social media boundaries

Social media is part of most of our lives now. How much you allow it into your life can influence your well-being and therefore your mental health.

Social media has contributed to lack of confidence, anxiety, self-loathing, eating disorders, depression and many other mental health issues. Love it or loathe it, social media is here to stay.

I have lost touch with the number of social media platforms available to join. It can be a superb way to hook up with people and make new contacts. I use it for my work and to connect with other writers. However, on a personal level, I am conscious of the connections I form and the interactions I have.

There is a lot of false information on the internet. This information can create fear, frustration and anger. As the various platforms fail to create appropriate boundaries to ensure that our well-being is not damaged, then it is up to each of us individually to do so.

Below is a list of general rules and guidelines I have set myself to ensure that I stay healthy and not damaged or stressed by social media.

- Only accept friend requests from people you know or who you are confident are 'genuine people' with whom you want to connect.

- Bear in mind that whatever you post is open to a negative comment or counter-argument. If in doubt then do not post.

- You can 'unfollow', 'de-friend' or 'block' anyone at any time. In particular, if you find someone is negative towards you or pulls your mood down.

- Do not get into debates and arguments. They tend to cause stress.

- Limit time on social media. It drains energy and well-being.

- Whatever you post is out for all to see, even if you delete it. It is often better not to post if you are very upset or reacting hastily. Give thought to posts and remember that others can misinterpret your sentiment sometimes.

- Do not go on social media after 8pm or before you have been up for an hour.

- Social media should be a positive experience. If it is not, then stop using it.

- Be conscious of what and who you connect with e.g. by 'liking' or 'commenting' on posts. Because of algorithms you are likely to get more of the same come through your newsfeed.

- Keep it positive, fun or informative.

- Do not use social media as a platform for moaning because it only keeps you in the negative.

- If you send a private message to someone and they do not respond immediately or are brief in their response, read nothing into this. There could be many reasons. Do not take it personally.

- Likewise, if you do not want to respond to a message straight away, that is fine too.

- Turn off any noise notifications so you are not constantly checking the platforms you are connected with every time they ping. This can be very distracting, counter-productive and create additional stress hormones.

Social media can be a great place to connect, learn new things, have a laugh, meet like-minded people and contact old or distant friends and family. However, it can also be a very unhealthy place if not suitably managed.

When using social media, consider its impact on your mental health. If there are any elements which are unhealthy or negative please make adjustments. I have known people decide to come off platforms altogether or to limit to 'viewing only' type applications, where there is no or little interaction, in a bid to look after their mental health.

Social media should be a positive experience. Create your own boundaries to protect your mental health.

40. Use your inner voice wisely

We all have an inner voice. In fact, you could say, we all have a number of inner voices.

When someone experiences mental health challenges, the inner voice is usually negative and goes through various scenarios of what might happen; the 'what ifs'. It also puts them down, telling them they are useless or cannot achieve certain things. The inner voice can ruin your day. If not controlled, it can help to ruin your enjoyment of life.

The inner voice is based on many things. In particular:

- Your belief system
- Learned behaviour (e.g. a parent always worrying may cause you to over worry too. Likewise, being frequently 'put down' could cause you to put yourself down as a matter of habit.)
- Life experiences
- The condition of your mental health
- Your own confidence and self-esteem
- The type of people you have mixed with. Negative people often offload their negativity onto you. Likewise, positive people can help you to see things more positivity.

The inner voice is the noise in your mind. It does not define or control you unless you allow it to. As you start to become more aware of these thoughts, observing them as a third party, you will begin to detach yourself from such negative and unhelpful thoughts. You will recognise them for what they are; the noise in your head and not the truth. You will no longer identify with that negativity. Instead, you will form a new, more positive and wonderful reality. This will mean that 'you' start to control your inner voice.

The quality of the inner voice can have a big impact on how we feel about ourselves, other people, activities and life in general. If we keep telling ourselves we are useless, pathetic or hopeless we are going to believe it, as it is the most overpowering information entering our mind.

It is important to address your inner voice so that you are talking positively about yourself and about what to expect from your day. Firstly, we need to know what your inner voice is like. Here are a few questions to help decide:

- Is your inner voice mostly positive or negative?
- Does it put you down?
- Does it remind you of someone else (e.g. a parent or teacher)?
- Does it worry a lot?
- Does it expect the worst to happen?
- Do you wish it would stop talking sometimes?

Usually when someone suffers with mental health problems, the inner voice is negative, worries a lot and expects bad things to happen. Very often it is self-critical too.

Here are a few examples of what the inner voice might be saying:

- What if that happens?
- I'm hopeless
- I can't do it
- I need to pull myself together
- I can't cope
- It's a disaster

- I'm pathetic
- I'm weak
- Everyone else is more successful than me

Years ago, I recognised my inner voice could sometimes be negative towards me. For example, if I dropped a glass, I would call myself "an idiot" or worse. I started to counter-act the negativity by saying "it's okay, everyone drops things, it's not the worst thing that could happen". My inner voice conversation would go something like this:

(Drop glass)
"You idiot" - my programmed response
"It's ok, these things happen. It's not a major disaster" – this phrase immediately diluted the first response and took some of the negative energy out of it.

As time went on and I continued this process, I recognised I was being more positive about myself:

(Drop glass)
"These things happen. It's no big deal. Let it go."
-The End-

The important point here is that I had stopped calling myself an 'idiot'! The programmed response had been phased out because it received no attention.

The more often you connect with the inner voice by using it in a positive way, the more automatic positive behaviour becomes. I also started to cut out negativity about simple things, such as the weather or being stuck at traffic lights.

"You're braver than you believe stronger than you seem and smarter than you think."

Alan Alexander Milne
Author

Important exercise

A simple exercise is to put an identity to the negative inner voice. Let's start with the voice that puts you down. For clarity, I will call this the self-negative voice.

1. Consider what the 'self-negative voice' looks like. Give it a visual identity such as a clown, an animal, a person, a comedy character; anything you wish.
2. Then create a name for the 'self-negative voice'.
3. Finally, what does it sound like? Is it a wobbly voice, a soft voice, a squeaky voice? It might sound like your normal voice.

So now you have a visual identity, a name and you recognise the sound of the self-negative voice.

For my example, I have Domino the Devil, who sounds snippy, behind my self-negative voice.

Now you need a more encouraging and positive character. They could remind you of someone you know, perhaps a friend, relative or colleague. Do the same process for this character.

1. Consider what the 'encouraging and positive voice' might look like. Give it a visual identity such as a panther, a superhero, an actor, anything you wish.

2. Then consider what the name of this 'encouraging and positive voice' would be.
3. Finally, what does it sound like? Is it a strong voice, a relaxed voice, a confident voice? It may sound like a person you know who is encouraging, confident and positive.

I am going to use a character one of my clients came up with, which is brilliant, the actor Will Smith. I am not sure I could think of someone more smiley and positive.

Here's what you do next:

Every time the self-negative voice fires up, so in my case Domino the Devil, with those worry thoughts, Will Smith is going to jump in with a new, more positive, perspective. Here are some examples:

Domino the Devil:	*"I will never get a promotion. I'm not cut out for management."*
Will Smith:	*"I am very capable. I will prove myself and get that promotion."*
Domino the Devil:	*"I am not as capable or confident as other guys."*
Will Smith:	*"I am going to learn new skills and give new things a try. I am just as capable as everyone else."*

Domino the Devil:	*"I could never run a marathon. I am so unfit."*
Will Smith:	*"I am going to read up on running and follow a training schedule so I can build up my fitness. In two years' time I will run a marathon."*

From the examples above, you can see just how important our inner voice is.

When you start to open your mind to another perspective, a more encouraging and confident perspective, you realise your inner voice has been lying to you. It has been over focusing on the negatives, causing you to believe them and has not been allowing positive thoughts or comments from others in. The truth has become blurred in the process.

Your inner voice has been completely unjust and unfair to you. It's been limiting you and holding you back. It has been unkind and now is the right time to balance things out.

The inner voice requires a little effort on your part but soon you will see a more balanced and honest view. You will start to recognise and question some of your negative thoughts. Then you will add the positivity and take control of your inner voice.

Use your positive and encouraging inner voice because you are listening.

41. Visualise what you do want

Visualisation is a beneficial tool in helping you in many ways. The subconscious mind works very well with the imagination. There is no requirement to be a strong visualiser. I am not a great visualiser but when I use this technique, it helps me with my goals.

Without being aware of it, we use imagery via the subconscious mind throughout the day. This might be recalling previous events or considering future scenarios.

We are constantly flicking through visual imagery, either of the past, or of a future we expect or desire. Usually when people experience mental health problems, there is a strong visualisation focus towards the past which then impacts the present and the future.

Old memories are etched into the subconscious mind. For this reason, you are receiving constant, albeit often unconscious, reminders of the bleak times from your past. You then apply this information towards future situations.

Someone who suffers anxiety will be visualising many types of possible negative scenarios into their future, which are often based on previous experiences.

Visualisation is one of the most beneficial tools in helping to create a successful, confident, happy and healthy mindset. We therefore need to plant some positive visual seeds in order to create a better future.

To start with, we shall get you in tune with your imagination. Sit comfortably, away from distraction, as you are about to picture a scene. Take your time with this exercise, pausing at the different images, so you can tune into the scene:

'You are walking along a beach in your bare feet. Be aware of the feel of the soft dry sand underfoot and beneath your toes. You can hear seagulls in the distance. The sky is clear blue and the sun is beaming down on you. There is a slight swell and you watch the water lapping against the shore. There are just a few other people on the beach. You notice a couple walking their small dog. The dog is having fun around the water's edge. A family are sat on some rocks and two children are playing in rock pools. There is a gentle warm breeze against your face, it feels pleasant. Here you feel very calm and peaceful. Your mind is calm.'

Take a moment to read through the visualisation once or twice more, then close your eyes and imagine the scene. Take plenty of time to get into the zone. You can add any other elements to the visualisation you desire.

Along with the skill of visualisation, the above exercise also includes kinaesthetic (feel) elements, i.e. 'the soft dry sand underfoot and beneath your toes'. Sound is another aspect, 'you can hear the seagulls in the distance'. Of the five senses, there are three primary senses, namely visual, kinaesthetic and auditory. The remaining two are taste and smell. Some people will be more strongly connected to one of these five senses. If you are more kinaesthetic, for example, you will gain more from connecting with feelings and sensations. If you are mostly auditory focused, you will be drawn in by sounds.

Do not concern yourself with how strongly you see imagery.

Just by using your imagination, you are making important connections and your subconscious mind will make those all-important changes.

There are several ways you can use visualisation.

Positive experiences

Making a connection with positive experiences can be a great benefit. These can be actual events from your past or imagined events. This is best achieved by letting the memories (or imagined events) come to mind, rather than trying to force them through.

In order to guide your mind a little, here is an introduction. Take your time pondering on the following:

There are many events stored in your very wonderful subconscious mind. Some you will have remembered, others forgotten to your conscious mind. There is that very first memory. This may be a family event or perhaps your first day at school. Did the home you grew up in have a garden or backyard? I wonder what you recall about those early years of your life? Was there a big gathering of some sort or the day it rained or snowed heavily? What do you recollect about the first day in your first job? How did you feel that day? Were you nervous or excited? A memory where you were spending time with your best friend. An achievement of some sort comes to mind. A special friendship or your first kiss, perhaps.

There are many memories stored in the subconscious mind. Some may have begun to rise to the surface already.

Now allow a positive memory to come to mind and spend a few moments associating with that memory. Where were you? Who was there? What was happening? How did you feel? Connect again with those good feelings. Allow yourself to feel those pleasant sensations once again. These might be joy, pride, peace, love or some other positive feelings. Notice where in your body you experience those good feelings.

You are meant to feel good. Over the days, weeks and months ahead you will experience more of these pleasant feelings as you continue to connect with good memories or create your own positive visualisations.

Repeat the above for a further four different events. If you cannot bring to mind good memories, then create your own scene of a place you would like to be, people you would be with and feelings you wish to feel. This would be similar to a daydream.

Alternatively, you could create a visualisation of something you wish to achieve in the future. Imagine being successful and all the good thoughts and feelings that come with this.

My favourite thing about the subconscious mind is that it does not differentiate between a real or created event. It accepts both types of events as real. This means you can use your imagination very powerfully to create positive change.

Future life

How do you want your future life to be? If you were to experience life the way you want to with self-belief, confidence, self-worth and pleasant feelings, what would that be like? Imagine where you would be, who you would be with and what you would be doing. This might be in relation to work, social or personal life.

If other aspects of your life were good such as your career, family life, home, hobbies and friendships, what would that look, sound and feel like? Take a few moments to explore a positive future. Use as many senses as possible.

If you do this frequently, then you are giving your mind useful direction. You are providing it with the blueprint for everything you want to bring into your life.

Calm scene

When we are not feeling good, it is helpful to create a scene that would put us into a good place, similar to the beach scene described above. Consider for a moment, where you feel most at peace. It could be a living room with a log fire, candles and some soothing music in the background, or walking through a meadow, hearing the birds sing, watching rabbits hop around and breathing in the fresh country air. You might recall a holiday destination which was especially peaceful and relaxing. Your calming scene can be anywhere you want it to be. It can be an actual place or a place you imagine.

Spend as long as you wish but at least 5 minutes in your calming scene, whether you are lying, sitting or walking. Use as many senses as possible to connect with your calming scene.

Summary

Please do not underestimate the power of the imagination. It serves many purposes. Through the imagination you can engage with positive emotions. Use the inspiration to guide your mind towards future successes or the life you wish to have. By doing so, you are sending useful information through to your subconscious, setting a blueprint for success. It is important to keep practicing visualisation to gain the greatest benefit.

Use your imagination to create the life and feelings you want.

Keep visualising in the most positive sense.

42. Create the life you desire

When people suffer with mental health issues, especially depression, they spend a lot of time thinking about the past. This may include things they have done, comments made to them, terrible events, awful actions against them and so on. By doing so, this is a constant reminder that life is not good and there is no joy to be had.

To change life for the better, it helps to know what we do want. Consider the following, assuming life was as you want it to be:

- How would you feel?
- Who would you spend your time with?
- What career would you be doing?
- Where would you live?
- What hobbies would you engage in?
- What would bring you joy?

You may not have the answers to these questions yet but these are important areas to consider.

To achieve some of the above, you might need to take important action. For example, if you wish to change career, you may need to study or re-train. You might want to purchase your own property or move somewhere else. This could require some long-term planning.

Whether you know all the answers to the above questions or not, there is benefit in daydreaming because this sets your creative mind in motion.

On many levels, your present situation might be good and you have everything you could hope for in terms of career, family and finances. In which case, you may wish to focus on removing the restraints of the past and building up more self-belief and confidence.

Take a moment to focus on a specific area which you know needs to change, even if at the moment you do not know how to make that adjustment. For example, let's consider that you need to change career.

We will use a technique called the Disney Strategy. This was inspired by Walt Disney and later developed by Robert Dilts in 1994. This strategy enables you to consider many options with no limitations. It will bring awareness and action into what is possible.

The Disney Strategy was based on three key components, the dreamer, the realist and the critic. Consider these three characters for a moment:

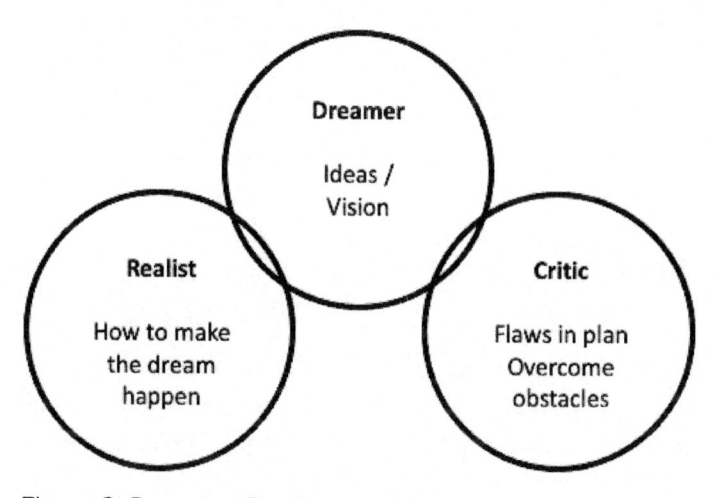

Figure 2. Dreamer, Realist and Critic.

The Dreamer

There are no boundaries or limitations to the Dreamer. They dream about what could be possible and, in their mind, anything is achievable. The Dreamer is full of passion about what could happen. They are enthusiastic and a complete optimist. They are open to any possibility. As the Dreamer, you throw all your ideas into the circle and disregard nothing at this stage. The Dreamer suggests a variety of options. Allow the creativity to flow. Be the ultimate optimist.

The Realist

The Realist's aim is to put the dream into action. They will sift through the options which are feasible and drop off those which are absolutely not possible.

For example, if the dreamer had considered being a firefighter but was 50 years old, this is most likely too old so you would strike this off the list. If, however, you were 20 years old, then the Realist can start to consider what action you can take to achieve this such as getting fit, taking your driving test and finding out about the tests to become a firefighter. The Realist is positive and solution-focussed.

The Critic

The Critic's job is to check for problems to the goal and plan. This might mean striking off more possibilities from the Dreamer's list to narrow the options down. The Critic will consider what is wrong with the idea or the steps proposed by the Realist to get there.

They are looking for flaws in the plan so they can consider

how to overcome any obstacles. You could consider them the pessimist but with a twist in that they will also be solution-focused. They find a flaw and then consider solutions to overcome it. It is only when there is no solution to be found that the idea is thrown out.

When using the Disney Strategy, you can imagine putting on a different hat for each character. It can also help to sit in a different place for each personality. If you struggle to get into role, think of someone you know or a fictitious character with each of the above traits.

You can take each idea in turn to go through the Realist and then Critic stages or you can take your preferred Dreamer idea first and move through the other stages. This would then look something like the example in Figure 3.

I have selected firefighter from the Dreamer list of ideas. I have then pursued this through the stages of Realist and Critic.

At the end of this process, you will have either a definitive option to pursue or several options which you can narrow down further.

You can use this same process for other matters such as moving to a house in the country or taking up a challenge. This process helps you to consider more options, use your creative mind more freely, create a solution-focused approach to life and explore possibilities. It is a great process for paving out a more positive future and problem solving.

Brainstorm ideas and take action to create the life you desire.

Have a solution-focussed mindset.

Dreamer

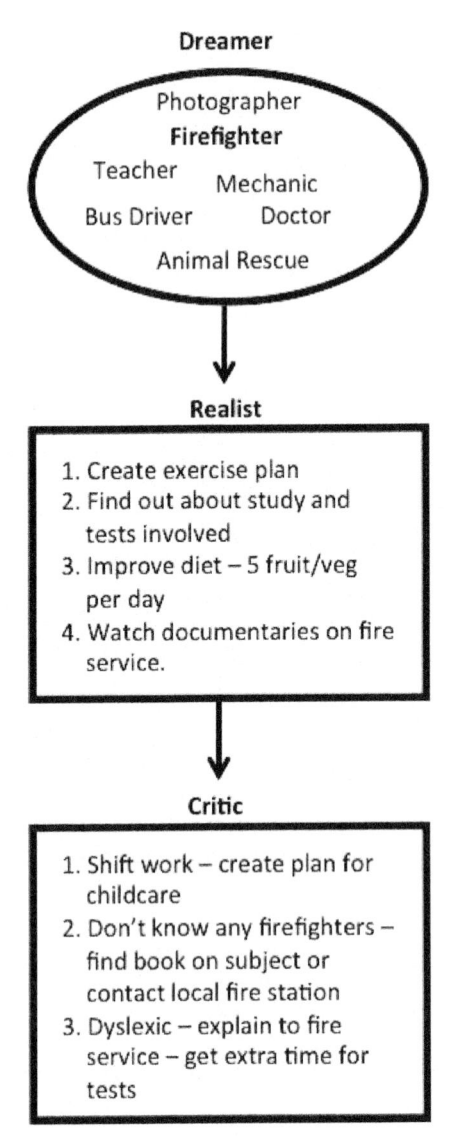

- Photographer
- **Firefighter**
- Teacher
- Mechanic
- Bus Driver
- Doctor
- Animal Rescue

Realist

1. Create exercise plan
2. Find out about study and tests involved
3. Improve diet – 5 fruit/veg per day
4. Watch documentaries on fire service.

Critic

1. Shift work – create plan for childcare
2. Don't know any firefighters – find book on subject or contact local fire station
3. Dyslexic – explain to fire service – get extra time for tests

Figure 3. Disney Strategy

43. Appreciate you

Usually when people struggle with mental health issues, they feel bad about themselves. They are often derogatory about many aspects, such as their personality, the way they look, the mistakes they have made and regrets. They dismiss their talents, skills and achievements. Mental health challenges cause people to focus on all the negatives they see in themselves and remind them of these over and over.

If you are doing this, you are giving yourself an unfair view of yourself. You would never be so hard on a friend, so why treat yourself in such a negative way? This has to change.

This exercise is to help you appreciate your qualities. I should let you know that, although it appears a straightforward exercise, many people struggle with it because they are so down on themselves. It can be beneficial to ask someone to help you with this; a person who knows you well and will encourage and support you.

I have created a 'self-recognition form' at the back of this book for you to complete for this exercise.

Exercise

Consider how your life will be when you feel good. Take yourself into the future. This is a positive future. Complete the following sentences. Supply three answers for each question, even if you need to return later to complete this exercise.

- When I feel good I will........(e.g. change jobs, spend more time with friends, join a choir).
- When I feel good, my life will be different because....(e.g.

I will gain enjoyment from life, I will believe in myself).
- When I feel good, I will see..... (e.g. people smiling, more people around me).
- When I feel good, I will hear..... (e.g. positive self-talk, laughter).

Now consider what needs to change for you to feel good. For example, I need to:

- take time for well-being activities
- be kinder to myself
- forgive myself
- believe in myself
- focus on the now
- visualise a positive future
- appreciate my achievements
- do more exercise
- accept compliments
- reduce social media time
- speak up for myself
- ignore negative comments from others
- accept myself for all my quirks and flaws
- create healthy habits
- remove negative people from my life

The time has come to recognise and appreciate the many great attributes you hold and offer. My guess is that until now, you have been far too tough on yourself and failed to appreciate all the great things you have achieved, are capable of and, of course, your superb personality traits.

Some people feel embarrassed to appreciate their successes and all the wonderful aspects about themselves. However, it is important to get over this. We do not need to be brash about it but can certainly acknowledge what we have achieved and our best bits. Let's call this modest acknowledgement.

I would like you to make a note of five of your best personality traits. You can get some help with this but you must acknowledge and agree with the five you decide on. Consider, what people appreciate you for? Are you the one they contact when they want a listening ear or the one who makes everyone laugh?

I am listing some examples of my own, to give you a flavour for this.

- Determined
- Speak my mind
- Authentic
- Excellent sense of humour
- Stand up for the underdog

Sometimes it can be fun asking a variety of people who know you well to list what they see as your best personality traits.

Next, consider what skills and abilities do you hold? These do not need to be complex or rare. Throughout life we absorb many skills and abilities yet ignore or dismiss them as unimportant, irrelevant or unimpressive. Here is my list of five:

- I can ski
- I'm good with animals (especially cats)
- I can write in a way that many people relate to
- I'm good at creating solutions
- I can drive a gearbox kart

Just to give the above some context; I can ski any run, including black runs and moguls, but I am not an outstanding skier. However, it is still a skill/ability I have. You do not need to be the best to acknowledge what you are capable of.

Next, what are five achievements you have attained over the course of your life so far? These can be from any time in your life. Here are mine:

- Built my own house
- Passed my driving test
- Run my own therapy practice
- Learned shorthand
- Wrote and published my first book

These need not be extraordinary achievements. It is, however, important that you give yourself recognition for your successes no matter how grand or small they are. This may be about getting a job or passing an exam of some sort. Perhaps you have won an award. You will have achieved far more than you give yourself credit for and will hold more skills and talents than you care to mention.

Acknowledge all the wonderful things about yourself.

You are incredible, capable and brilliantly you!

44. Positive tapping

Tapping was a technique introduced by Gary Craig to clear emotion and negative beliefs, which is still its primary use. However, variations of the technique have been developed. A useful way to use this technique for yourself is a method I call positive tapping.

Tapping points

To start with, you should get used to the tapping points. These are highlighted on Figure 4.

The tapping points in sequence is:

Karate chop (side of hand)
Top of head (nearer the back)
Eyebrow (where it starts)
Side of eye (follow eye socket)
Under eye (follow eye socket)
Under nose
Chin/under lip (where we have an indent)
Under collarbone
Under arm (in line with the nipple for men)
Side of thumb (alongside the nail)
Side of index finger
Side of middle finger
Side of ring finger
Side of little finger

Use positive tapping to focus on the change you desire, i.e. how you want to feel or what will benefit you as a belief. There is no limitation to what you can use the positive tapping for. You can focus on confidence, happiness, motivation or

Stresses of Modern Man

EFT Tapping Points

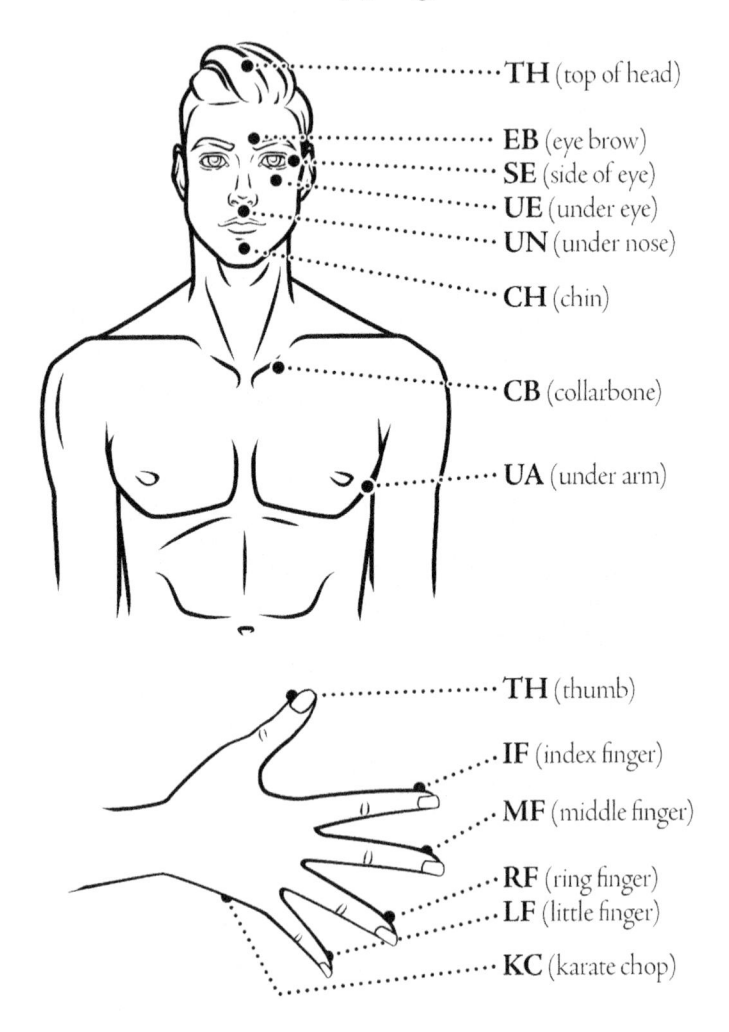

- **TH** (top of head)
- **EB** (eye brow)
- **SE** (side of eye)
- **UE** (under eye)
- **UN** (under nose)
- **CH** (chin)
- **CB** (collarbone)
- **UA** (under arm)
- **TH** (thumb)
- **IF** (index finger)
- **MF** (middle finger)
- **RF** (ring finger)
- **LF** (little finger)
- **KC** (karate chop)

Figure 4. Emotional Freedom Technique tapping points.

self-esteem for example. It is best to focus on one key issue at a time. This ensures you give it your full attention.

I tap quite softly and fairly quickly. It certainly should not be painful or uncomfortable. Tapping on some of the eye points can cause people to have a mini-reflex jolt until they are used to them, although this is less likely if you are tapping on yourself. I do not tap for a set number of taps, just as long as it takes me to say each phrase.

Spend a few days tapping through these points until you can tap without the need to refer to the book or diagram.

When you are ready move onto the wording.

It is helpful to write down a few thoughts, focusing on how you want to feel and what would be useful for you to believe.

I have prepared a number of scripts for you to try out. Below is one example. Further examples covering different scenarios are included under the Appendix section.

Before you start the tapping, it can be helpful to score the issue from 0-10. How high out of 10 do you consider your level of self-acceptance to be? The closer to ten suggests that it is less of a problem for you. The lower the score, the more of a problem it is. Therefore, if you score 2/10, this would suggest that your struggle with self-acceptance. The higher the score, the higher the self-acceptance. Then, check-in after each round of tapping to see if the score has changed.

Script 1. Tapping for self-acceptance

Karate chop: **I fully accept myself**
Karate chop: **I am a good person**
Karate chop: **I choose to believe in myself**

Now on through the other points:

Top of head: **I have skills and abilities**
Eyebrow: **I do my best in every situation**
Side of eye: **I fully accept myself**
Under eye: **I am a good person**
Under nose: **I choose to believe in myself**
Chin/under lip: **I have skills and abilities**
Collarbone: **I do my best in every situation**
Under arm: **I fully accept myself**

Thumb: **I am a good person**
Index finger: **I choose to believe in myself**
Middle finger: **I have skills and abilities**
Ring finger: **I do my best in every situation**
Little finger: **I fully accept myself**

Take a deep breath and have a sip of water. Ideally do this after each round of tapping.

Check-in:

How did that feel for you? Was it comfortable or difficult? If it was challenging, this suggests there is something held within your subconscious which needs to clear in this script for you.

What is the current score for self-acceptance? Has there been a change?

Did you notice any physical sensations? You can tap through these in the next round. For example, butterflies in the chest or tightness in the throat. The physical sensations represent the change in energy in your physical body as you release the underlying issue. These will clear as you clear the emotion.

Were there any sticking points where you experienced a wave of emotion? Emotion is a good response to tapping. It means that you are clearing out the negatives and releasing them.

We release emotion, negative beliefs and subconscious blockages in different ways when tapping. Sometimes through feelings and sensations, other times through words, yawning, tears, even belching and stomach grumbles. Sometimes a massive wave of emotion washes over you and the result of this is a powerful release. Go with the flow.

You may hold a strong belief, which makes it difficult for you to say some phrases. When this happens, the words will just not come out of your mouth no matter how hard you try.

If you do struggle to say a phrase, it would suggest that you do not believe the words you were trying to say at a subconscious level. That phrase does not agree with your belief system and understanding of reality. An example phrase could be "I'm a good person". You may believe very strongly that you are a bad person. This stops you saying those words. There will be subconscious blockages to clear. If you struggle to get some words out, I suggest you use another phrase. In which case you could say "I sometimes do good things" or "I have good aspects to my personality" or "others say I am a good person, I am open to believing that I am"

If you struggle to say "I fully accept myself" change this to "I am open to fully accepting myself" or "I wish to fully accept myself". You might find after a few rounds of this revised wording, you can then say the original phrase. This suggests you are making progress.

Going back to the script. Do you feel the need to do another round of tapping with the same wording? Alternatively, would you like to move on to different wording related to something else that comes to mind? When it comes to another round of tapping trust your intuition. If in doubt, do another two or three rounds with the original wording from Script 1.

Here is an example of how you might do another round with some feedback on Script 1. I have underlined any changes or new phrases based on hypothetical feedback being:

a) I found it hard to say: **I fully accept myself**
b) I have a: **feeling in my stomach - like butterflies**
c) I have a: **memory of bullying**

Onto the next round of tapping. Personalise for yourself as much as you can.

Script 1 with feedback. Tapping for self-acceptance

Karate chop: **I <u>am open to</u> fully accepting myself**
Karate chop: **I am a good person**
Karate chop: **I choose to believe in myself**

Now on through the other points:

Top of head: **<u>These butterflies in my stomach</u>**

Eyebrow: **I do my best in every situation**
Side of eye: **I am open to fully accepting myself**
Under eye: **This memory of bullying**
Under nose: **These butterflies in my stomach**
Chin/under lip: **I have skills and abilities**
Collarbone: **I do my best in every situation**
Under arm: **This memory of bullying**

Thumb: **I am a good person**
Index finger: **I choose to believe in myself**
Middle finger: **I have skills and abilities**
Ring finger: **This memory of bullying**
Little finger: **I am open to fully accepting myself**

Check in again and continue with the tapping.

It is possible that you would benefit from additional support or more specific tapping to help release memories. More information and options for tapping are contained in my earlier books, *The Energy of Anxiety* and *The Power of Confidence*.

You may also wish to consider working with an EFT practitioner upon reviewing the 'Therapy Options' section if Tapping is something you are open to pursuing.

Take a look in the Appendix for further scripts. It will take a while to get used to tapping but it is worth persevering.

Select a positive tapping script and start to make progress by clearing subconscious blockages and lingering emotions.

45. Three words tapping

Using the three words tapping is a great way to get used to the points and the process. During my days of competitive cycling, I used three key words, which became mantras. I then combined these with tapping. I would go through between three and six rounds of tapping, using my three words, before races. As I found this helpful, I suggested this process to clients for certain issues and situations. People like it because of its simplicity.

Here's how it works. Consider three keywords that will help you connect with what you want to experience. For example, you may wish to feel *calm*, *confident* and *peaceful*. I will use these as an example for this tapping exercise.

Spend some time each day doing a few rounds of tapping and, as you go through the points, keep repeating the words.

You can also use these words with sneaky tapping by imagining tapping on the points and saying the words inside your mind. Alternatively, just tap on the finger points using the thumb of the same hand. Most people will not notice you doing this and those who do will just think you are fiddling. I realise most people are self-conscious about tapping and do not want to be seen tapping on the top of their head or around the face in public. This is why the sneaky tapping is helpful.

At times you can also use the three words without the tapping, so they become your mantras.

With the three-word tapping, we miss out the karate chop point and go straight to the top of the head.

As you tap, you say the relevant word.

> Top of head - **Calm**
> Eyebrow - **Confident**
> Side of eye - **Peaceful**
> Under eye - **Calm**
> Under nose - **Confident**
> Chin/under lip - **Peaceful**
> Under collarbone - **Calm**
> Under arm - **Confident**
> Thumb - **Peaceful**
> Index finger - **Calm**
> Middle finger - **Confident**
> Ring finger - **Peaceful**
> Little finger - **Calm**

This completes one round. Do at least three rounds of tapping, although you can do more. I suggest doing this daily for three weeks in order that the process becomes second nature for you. The best times to do this are in the morning, not long after awakening, and before you go to bed at night. It will take you just a minute or two to do.

Because you can do sneaky tapping, you can use this technique at any time. Also remember, you can use the words as mantras without the tapping.

I prefer people to stick to the same three words so you build a powerful connection with them. However, if you later decide that other words suit you better, you can change them. You can draw upon your three words easily, once you have practiced this regularly, even in stressful situations. You may also want to have a different set of three words for specific situations but try not to over complicate the process,

Stresses of Modern Man

certainly in the early stages.

For ease of reference, I am listing below a number of possible three-word combinations but it is important for you to use words which you connect with.

Self-belief/confidence
Believe - Confident - I will

Calm
Calm - Peaceful - Breathe
(As you say 'breathe' take a deep breath)

Focus
Focused - Clear - Observant

Self-acceptance
Kindness - Self-love - Appreciation

Positivity
Joy - Happiness - Gratitude

Decide which subject will help you to benefit the most from the three words tapping. Do at least three rounds in the morning and the evening. You can do more at any time in the day.

Use the Three-Words Tapping every day to create a positive attitude towards yourself and life.

46. Mental health plan

It can be helpful to monitor how you are feeling each day. It is also going to help your progress to do well-being activities regularly and keep focused on a healthy lifestyle. The form below will help you to keep track of this.

Remember, this is a guide. We are not seeking perfection and you will not always progress. In the early days you may still have more down days than good days but over time, you will begin to have more good days. The form will help you recognise trends and where you are going off-track. It acts as a reminder to do the various activities and have self-awareness.

If you forget to complete the form for a day or two, do not worry or be hard on yourself, just pick it up where you are now.

If you are seeing a therapist, you may wish to use the form as a reference point to provide updates.

I have included an example completed copy of this form under the Appendix section. You can go to my website www.abauthor.com for downloadable forms.

Score 1 = low or poor
Score 5 = high or great

Sleep Quality (1-5)		Sleep Hours	
Morning Mood (1-5)		Healthy snacks ✓✗	
Breakfast ✓✗		Water (litres)	
Energy after breakfast (1-5)		Working Hours	

Lunch ✓✗		Energy during day (1-5)	
Dinner ✓✗		Afternoon/Evening Mood (1-5)	
Exercise Type		Exercise Duration	
Affirmations Repeated (number)		Gratitudes (number)	

Therapist session notes

Well-being activities

Worries

Social contact (e.g. friends/family)

Highs and lows

Positive visualisation - goal/notes

EFT - positive/3 words - what was focus for tapping?

Unhealthy activities e.g. alcohol, smoking etc

What made you feel bad/why?

What made you feel good/why?

Notes for the day

Complete the mental health plan daily to keep on track.

Regular completion will help you notice what causes problems and what benefits you.

47. Therapy options

Before I go through therapy options, please remember that the following is based on my opinions, skillset and knowledge from working with my clients.

In writing this book, I pondered how best to help without over-burdening you with information or techniques.

By using the exercises and taking the advice in this book, you will benefit. How much you benefit is down to how severe your mental health issues are to start with, what stresses you are dealing with now and how committed you are to the exercises and making lifestyle improvements.

You might find that you have learned all you need through this book and within a few weeks or month are back to being in a good place, which would be fantastic. Having said that, everyone is different. Each person's life experiences are unique. Therefore, only time will tell how far and how quickly you progress.

If you are struggling moderately to severely with your mental health, I encourage you to seek professional help.

Having therapy to overcome mental health issues can be more beneficial than you might appreciate right now. It is not always the obvious type of treatment that provides the greatest benefit. When people think of therapy, they imagine being sat in a chair across from a psychotherapist who is holding a clipboard, rubbing their chin as they analyse their client. The therapist is asking awkward questions and the client is being asked to go into great detail about the problems in their life. They feel extremely uncomfortable and self-conscious. However, I have good news for you, this does not have to be the case.

With the right therapist you will feel at ease. It is not at all as scary or uncomfortable as you might imagine. You will not feel judged and will gain a sense that they want to help. There should not be a hierarchy feel to the session. You should feel comfortable with your therapist and the setting.

Excellent therapy depends on the following, in no particular order:

- A quality therapist.
- A good and suitable rapport with your therapist.
- Commitment to the process, i.e. attend sessions.
- Follow up with any suggestions for continued self-work between sessions.
- An open-minded approach. Be open to making progress.
- Feedback through the sessions.
- A client-specific approach (not one-size fits all).
- You must feel listened to and ensure that your unique circumstances are taken into account.
- You should feel at ease enough to discuss anything you want.

I have had significant success using a combination of my favoured therapies. These are Hypnotherapy, Matrix Reimprinting, Emotional Freedom Technique (EFT or Tapping) and Colour Mirrors. Resolution to problems happens on many levels, consciously, subconsciously, energetically and physically. The subconscious resolution is massively important. Remember, the subconscious mind is your programming centre.

When seeking to work with a professional, you may call upon friends and family to seek referrals. Most of my work comes via referrals. Sometimes it can be worth travelling to see a good therapist and, with modern technology, sessions can be conducted over the internet. This is something I do with clients who are not based where I live and it has worked very well. You need a suitable room from where to conduct your session, where you can be comfortable and will not be disturbed.

You can achieve so much through therapy and commitment to the process.

Insight into my therapies

I enjoy working with clients with mental health problems. This is partly because they are always great people. Also, I know we can make a big difference to their quality of life.

Behind successful therapy requires an ability to understand each individual, their challenges, their background and what has blocked them from achieving good mental health so far. Sometimes solutions require stepping outside of the box. Other times the solutions are simpler than you might imagine.

Here is a brief insight behind those therapies:

Hypnotherapy

Becoming relaxed, or being in a state of trance, enables a better connection with, and access to, the subconscious mind. There are many myths about hypnotherapy and the state of trance, so here is a little information to ensure you gain a better understanding:

- You maintain control throughout the session.
- When in the state of trance, you feel more relaxed than usual.
- Most people will maintain conscious awareness, i.e. you will know where you are and feel in control but more relaxed than usual.
- You are not asleep.
- You will hear your therapist.
- You do not have to remember everything said to you. Your subconscious will take care of this.
- Trance is a really pleasant state. It is similar to a meditative state.
- Just think of trance as being relaxed.
- People often get into this state easier with a little practice, once you know what to expect and are familiar with your surroundings.

I call the state of trance "turning off your stress button". It is a wonderful state to be in.

By being in this state, there are two significant benefits (1) you are more able to access information stored in your subconscious mind than you would in a more awakened and alert state; (2) you are in a more solution-focused state of mind, which allows helpful changes to occur.

Trance helps you understand personal blocks to success and make changes. This is a great state for inducing positivity. You can also create positive visualisations. There are a variety of helpful techniques using the mind, which work very well when in this more relaxed state.

The most important thing is that you should feel at ease with the hypnotherapist. If you do not, relaxing may be more difficult. In the unlikely event that this is the case, I suggest you find another therapist.

Emotional Freedom Technique (tapping)

Tapping has been shown to produce powerful results. Already, in this book, you have had an opportunity to use a couple of tapping options. There is so much to be explored with the use of tapping. When you work with a practitioner, they should be able to do the deeper work for you and you can continue to tap for yourself as you wish. Depending on how experienced you become, it is possible to work through many issues for yourself.

Mindfulness Based Inner RePatterning (MBIR)

MBIR was developed by Tania Prince and June Spencer. It is a combination of tapping, focused breathing and mindfulness. Mindfulness is a state of mind achieved by focusing one's awareness on the present moment whilst free of resistance.

It is a very useful technique if you do not wish to go into detail on issues to be addressed. It requires developing an awareness of what you are experiencing in the moment. Using MBIR, you are taken into a state of inner peace. Through focussing on a specific issue which is problematic to you, MBIR helps you to release it.

Matrix Reimprinting (Matrix)

Matrix is very close to being a combination of hypnotherapy and tapping. Developed by Karl Dawson, it has become a very successful therapy. This treatment is a technique that connects people with their past traumas. These traumas link with unhelpful core beliefs which get in the way of us leading the life we want. Through the process, emotions and the trauma are released.

Matrix works on three levels: the subconscious mind, the matrix of information all around us and your body's energy meridian system.

The basic root of Matrix is to tap on your 'younger self' or 'ECHO' to release a trauma. An ECHO is an 'energetic consciousness hologram'. You are helping your 'younger self' find resolution to the trauma.

This process releases the emotion and 'energy' of the event. You bring understanding about the incident. A new memory is then created, which helps to let go of any negative beliefs.

Matrix can be beneficial for the more challenging traumas and is best conducted under the guidance of a qualified practitioner, as some issues need to be handled with extreme care.

Colour Mirrors

Colour Mirrors is not a therapy in the conventional sense. Colour Mirrors is a system made from coloured oils and essences which are stored in bottles. This system was created by Melissie Jolly, a South African woman, who I look upon as incredibly wise and spiritual.

The word 'mirror' means a reflection of you, your life journey, emotions, experiences, what you are going through right now and many other aspects of you and your life.

This process works at a subconscious level and people are usually amazed at just how perfect the bottles they have chosen are to the issue being addressed. Each bottle has wording to reflect the energy of that bottle. This can be incredibly powerful and guide you to continue your journey of personal development.

In many ways the bottles offer something unique and special. The benefits from using Colour Mirrors can happen on many levels. In reality you have to experience them to fully appreciate what they are about.

I became interested in Colour Mirrors when these amazing bottles were used on me and, as I inhaled each essence, the negative emotions dissipated instantly. I was also amazed at how the wording for each individual bottle was so relevant to the issues I was addressing.

I love using the bottles as part of a therapy session or on their own either in a one-to-one session or a workshop. The Colour Mirrors are inspirational and carry so much wisdom. They help you release stress and trauma from your subconscious mind and body cells. They can bring understanding, clarity and can help you turn your life around.

I often get the sense that some guys wonder what they have walked into when they see the bottles in my studio. I will give them a brief overview of the bottles and explain how we might use them.

It has been known for them to be quite shocked at how the bottles have helped them to release trauma, stress or other blocks. Sometimes, we do not need to fully understand how something works to achieve success. In a way the Colour

Stresses of Modern Man

Mirrors provide intangible solutions. I have had so many amazing sessions with clients and witnessed great shifts. The wording also gives us new ways to view life and our experiences. That in itself is healing. Children absolutely love them too.

Rhythmic Movement Training international (RMTi)

RMTi is also not a therapy but a way of creating positive change on many levels. It is a process, which helps to integrate primitive and postural reflexes, which have either become active or never been integrated. This can be for a variety of reasons, including complications in the womb or during birth, illness, trauma, injury or missing vital developmental stages in the early years of life.

The Fear Paralysis Reflex and the Moro Reflex are two reflexes specifically related to anxiety. They are also considered to be linked to anxiety and emotional outbursts associated with ASD.

As a Consultant in RMTi, I have seen great improvements with my clients on many issues. RMTi is a movement-based approach which, over time, helps to build the brain connections needed to function well. This has to be conducted at a steady rate as building neurons is no small task. The rewards of RMTi can be invaluable.

In RMTi, the consultant assesses the client and then directs the process to make the connections within the brain. The client then continues to do the selected exercises at home and visits the consultant on a monthly basis (or as appropriate) to check on progress and decide on the next set of exercises.

RMTi can help behaviour, OCD, postural challenges,

co-ordination, ADD, ADHD, ASD, dyspraxia, dyslexia, anxiety, insecurity and many other issues.

In summary

I know the power of these therapies and I am passionate about what is possible. Of course, there are other therapeutic options you might wish to investigate. My experience suggests that few people overcome their mental health challenges without working with the subconscious mind because this is where our memories are stored and programming is set.

Success is heavily weighted on your connection with your practitioner. Moving away from tradition, many people are finding greater results by taking the holistic route rather than traditional therapies. When we are prepared to release what has been holding us back, so much is possible.

If you have a bad day or week, know something better is around the corner. Use the health plan to help you create that positive future and move away from anything which is not good for your well-being.

Please do not place limits on what you can change or achieve. Do not be restricted by any medical diagnosis or any limiting beliefs you held before reading this book.

I hope 'Stresses of Modern Man' has given you direction, encouragement and hope for the future.

With commitment you have a magnificent opportunity to free yourself of everything that has been holding you back. You have made it this far. Just imagine what is possible with some help and support.

48. My final message

I hope you have found this book both informative and useful. I encourage you to use the techniques and keep notes using the health plan form.

One of the important messages I want you to take from this book is, no matter what your mental health issue, you are not flawed. You are an exceptional and brilliant individual, who is capable and can achieve tremendous amounts. I want you to value yourself. It is important that you recognise your self-worth.

You are every bit as good as any other person. In fact, you are more amazing than most of us because you have endured so much and yet you are still here fighting to live a better life.

In reality, we are all doing our best given the challenges that happen in life and the knowledge we hold. Some people have more than their fair share of awful situations but, despite this, significant change is possible.

Mental health issues are, in most cases, a response to situations. Those situations can happen at any time in your life. Because mental health issues are mostly related to life events, this means there is great potential for you to overcome these challenges.

As you progress, occasionally you may have a setback. There will be days when you feel your mental health has gone backwards. Please do not be deterred by this as it is also part of the journey. Never let a setback stop you from striving to make changes and create a better life for yourself. You can do it.

Please remember what I have said about appreciating yourself. My guess is that you have been far too tough on yourself. Give yourself praise when you achieve something. Be gentle and kind to yourself. You deserve it.

Whatever you are going through right now, is part of your life's journey but you have not yet reached your final destination. There is plenty more to come and you can start directing your life in the way you want it go.

You may need to remove yourself from the company of some people who are negative or put you down. Perhaps you need to be more proactive with your wellness programme. You may know that you must build up your self-esteem, self-worth and self-confidence. This is a common theme in people who experience mental health difficulties.

Some days you will be more motivated to do the well-being activities than others. That is okay. Do not beat yourself up about what you do not do. Give yourself praise for what you do achieve though.

Remember that self-preservation is not selfishness. Sometimes you have to put yourself first to survive and create good health. This is important. Self-preservation is a necessity. It is non-negotiable.

Please appreciate yourself. Accept yourself for the person you are. Whatever the state of your health, acknowledge this is where you are now but does not have to be where you are heading.

I have witnessed many amazing people, who have struggled with their mental health, come out the other side to live an enjoyable and fulfilling life. This is achieved through commitment to change and the processes which help that to occur.

You are more capable than you realise and can make a start in changing your life for the better today.

Huge transformation is possible.

You have what it takes to live a better life.

All power to you.

I am by your side, willing you on, all of the way.

Appendix

I. Communication Form

Please complete as much information on this form as you feel able to and hand it to someone, in order to open up communication and take that first positive step. This can also be found on my website.

Name: _____

I have been struggling for ...... days/weeks/months/years.

I am specifically worried about:_____

_____

_____

_____

_____

I have strange thoughts such as:_____

_____

_____

_____

_____

Stresses of Modern Man

I can't stop thinking about:_____

_____

_____

_____

I have negative thoughts which include:_____

_____

_____

_____

I have some physical feelings which include:_____

_____

_____

_____

I am using some unhealthy coping mechanisms:_____

_____

_____

_____

I am experiencing the following (tick ✓ those appropriate):

Lack of motivation		Thoughts of "what's the point?"	
Trouble sleeping		Suicidal thoughts	
Constant worry/anxiety		Self-loathing	
Feeling low/depression		Nausea/vomiting	
Drink too much alcohol		Self-medicating with _____	
Addicted to _____		Self-doubt/lack of confidence	
Digestive problems		Grieving for (person/animal) _____	
Physical pain (where) _____.		Regrets about _____	
Financial worries		Bullying	

Stresses of Modern Man

Worries about work		Fear about _____	
Nightmares/Terrors		Regret	
Ill health		Other _____	

I feel I am _____

_____

_____

_____

Add any further information you feel will be useful_____

_____

_____

_____

_____

_____

II. Tapping scripts

Here are some additional tapping scripts. Feel free to change any wording so the scripts are better personalised for you.

Script 2. Tapping for general confidence

Karate chop: **I am capable and ready for success**
Karate chop: **I believe in my skills and abilities**
Karate chop: **I am more than good enough**

Top of head: **I believe in my skills and abilities**
Eyebrow: **I am more than good enough**
Side of eye: **I encourage myself every step of the way**
Under eye: **I am capable and ready for success**
Under nose: **I believe in my skills and abilities**
Chin/under lip: **I am more than good enough**
Collarbone: **I encourage myself every step of the way**
Under arm: **I am capable and ready for success**

Thumb: **I believe in my skills and abilities**
Index finger: **I am more than good enough**
Middle finger: **I encourage myself every step of the way**
Ring finger: **I am capable and ready for success**
Little finger: **I believe in myself**

Check-in

- Take a deep breath and have a sip of water.
- How did that feel for you?
- Did you notice any physical sensations?
- Were there any sticking points where you felt a wave of emotion?

- Did you find some phrases difficult to say?
- Did any memories come to mind?
- Do you feel the need to do another round with the same wording or would you like to move on to a round of tapping with new wording? Trust what feels right. If in doubt, do another two or three rounds using this current wording.

Utilise anything that you notice in future rounds of tapping. I will not continue to list the above check-in list but please continue to use it in order to help you assess how you are progressing or where there are any sticking points.

Script 3. Removing negativity from others

Karate chop: **I fully believe in myself**
Karate chop: **I activate my full potential**
Karate chop: **I am confident in my abilities**

Top of head: **I release negativity from others**
Eyebrow: **I am a good person**
Side of eye: **I release negativity from my mind and body**
Under eye: **If others are negative, the negativity belongs to them**
Under nose: **I fully believe in myself**
Chin/under lip: **I activate my full potential**
Collarbone: **I am confident in my abilities**
Under arm: **I release negativity from others**

Thumb: **I am a good person**
Index finger: **I release negativity from my mind and body**
Middle finger: **If others are negative, the negativity belongs to them**
Ring finger: **I fully believe in myself**
Little finger: **I release negativity from others**

Take a deep breath and have a sip of water.

Check-in.

Script 4. Creating a bright future

Karate chop: **I choose joy and happiness**
Karate chop: **I am joy and happiness**
Karate chop: **I'm creating a peaceful mind**

Top of head: **I have a bright future**
Eyebrow: **I believe in a happy future**
Side of eye: **I choose joy and happiness**
Under eye: **I am joy and happiness**
Under nose: **I'm creating a peaceful mind**
Chin/under lip: **I have a bright future**
Collarbone: **I believe in a happy future**
Under arm: **I choose joy and happiness**

Thumb: **I am joy and happiness**
Index finger: **I'm creating a peaceful mind**
Middle finger: **I have a bright future**
Ring finger: **Positivity is entering my life**
Little finger: **I embrace a bright future**

Take a deep breath and have a sip of water.

Check-in.

Script 5. Creating a positive day

Karate chop: **A new day offers new opportunities**
Karate chop: **I am grateful for all I have** (you can mention specific things you are grateful for)
Karate chop: **I see the positive in situations**

Top of head: **I grow through life experiences**
Eyebrow: **I seek out opportunities**
Side of eye: **Today is bright**
Under eye: **A new day offers new opportunities**
Under nose: **I am grateful for all I have**
Chin/under lip: **I see the positive in situations**
Collarbone: **I grow through life experiences**
Under arm: **I seek out opportunities**

Thumb: **Today is bright**
Index finger: **A new day offers new opportunities**
Middle finger: **I am grateful for all I have**
Ring finger: **I see the positive in situations**
Little finger: **I grow through life experiences**

Take a deep breath and have a sip of water.

Check-in.

Script 6. Creating calm

Karate chop: **I am safe**
Karate chop: **I am at peace**
Karate chop: **I am calm**

Top of head: **I am safe**
Eyebrow: **I am at peace**
Side of eye: **I am calm**
Under eye: **I am safe**
Under nose: **I am at peace**
Chin/under lip: **I am calm**
Collarbone: **I am safe**
Under arm: **I am at peace**

Thumb: **I am calm**
Index finger: **I am safe**
Middle finger: **I am at peace**
Ring finger: **I am calm**
Little finger: **I am safe**

Take a deep breath and have a sip of water.

Check-in.

Script 7. Releasing personal triggers

Karate chop: **I choose to release that which does not serve me**
Karate chop: **I release judgement on the behaviour of others**
Karate chop: **I release the expectations I have of others**

Top of head: **I connect with the energy of love**
Eyebrow: **I choose to release that which does not serve me**
Side of eye: **I release judgement on the behaviour of others**
Under eye: **I release the expectations I have of others**
Under nose: **I free myself of judgement**
Chin/under lip: **I connect with the energy of love**
Collarbone: **I choose to release that which does not serve me**
Under arm: **I release judgement on the behaviour of others**

Thumb: **I release the expectations I have of others**
Index finger: **I free myself of judgement**
Middle finger: **I am open to releasing all triggers**
Ring finger: **I am free and it feels good**
Little finger: **Thank you for bringing this issue to my attention so I can release it**

Take a deep breath and have a sip of water.

Check-in.

Script 8. Releasing anger

Karate chop: **Even though I feel angry, I choose to let it go**
Karate chop: **Even though I feel angry, I am ready to let it go**
Karate chop: **Even though I feel angry, I am empowered to let it go**

Top of head: **This anger**
Eyebrow: **Angry about............** (*mention the reason for the anger*)
Side of eye: **This tension in my jaw** (*or any other feelings you have*)
Under eye: **This tightness in my chest** (*or any other feelings you have*)
Under nose: **This anger**
Chin/under lip: **Angry about............** (*mention the reason for the anger*)
Collarbone: **This tension in my jaw** (*or any other feelings you have*)
Under arm: **This tightness in my chest** (*or any other feelings you have*)

Thumb: **I breathe out anger**
Index finger: **I breathe in calm**
Middle finger: **I am calm and relaxed**
Ring finger: **I choose to let it go**
Little finger: **I release all feelings of anger**

Take a deep breath and have a sip of water.

Check-in.

Script 9. Sleep script

Exclude the karate chop point. Do 3 - 6 rounds of this prior to bedtime.

Top of head: **Sleepy**
Eyebrow: **Peaceful**
Side of eye: **Calm**
Under eye: **Sleepy**
Under nose: **Peaceful**
Chin/under lip: **Calm**
Collarbone: **Sleepy**
Under arm: **Peaceful**

Thumb: **Calm**
Index finger: **Sleepy**
Middle finger: **Peaceful**
Ring finger: **Calm**
Little finger: **Sleepy**

If you awaken in the night, you can use the same three words and tap on the finger points using the thumb of the same hand. This can often be sufficient to release some tension and calm down the nervous system. Alternatively, just say the words inside your mind as you breathe deeply without the tapping.

Script 10. Let it go

This is a simple script when feeling any unwanted emotion. It's very useful for stress or anger. Do as many rounds as necessary to bring the emotion down. You can be more specific about the emotion and include any sensations you are feeling if you wish.

Exclude the karate chop point.

> Top of head: **Let it go**
> Eyebrow: **Let it go**
> Side of eye: **Let it go**
> Under eye: **Let it go**
> Under nose: **Let it go**
> Chin/under lip: **Let it go**
> Collarbone: **Let it go**
> Under arm: **Let it go**
>
> Thumb: **Let it go**
> Index finger: **Let it go**
> Middle finger: **Let it go**
> Ring finger: **Let it go**
> Little finger: **Let it go**

III. Example Health Plan

Score 1 = low or poor

Score 5 = high or great

Sleep Quality (1-5)	2	Sleep Hours	5
Morning Mood (1-5)	2	Healthy snacks ✓✗	✓
Breakfast ✓✗	✓	Water (litres)	2
Energy after breakfast (1-5)	3	Working Hours	7.5
Lunch ✓✗	✓	Energy during day (1-5)	3
Dinner ✓✗	✓	Afternoon/Evening Mood (1-5)	3
Exercise Type	Walk	Exercise Duration	40 mins
Affirmations Repeated (number)	6	Gratitudes (number)	3

Therapist session notes

Work on inner voice.

Stresses of Modern Man

Well-being activities *Soak in bath – 30 mins*
Worries *Too busy at work* *IBS will cause me problems*
Social contact (e.g. friends/family) *Colleagues – had brief chat at lunch time*
Highs and lows *Low – not enjoying work* *High – colleagues very understanding – felt justified in my concerns*
Positive visualisation - goal/notes *Doing a presentation at work confidently – ran through 3 times*
EFT - positive/3 words - what was focus for tapping? *3 words – calm, believe, relax*
Unhealthy activities e.g. alcohol, smoking etc *Smoking x 10*

What made you feel bad/why? *Work being so busy and feeling I can't cope*
What made you feel good/why? *Going for a walk. Colleagues being positive and helpful. Let person in queue behind me in shop go in front – made me feel good*
Notes for the day *I know work will calm down so just need to ride this busy period out. I can do it.*

IV. Self-recognition form

Complete this form to give you guidance on the life you want and appreciate yourself more.

Write down what life will be like when you feel good.

When I feel good I will _____

_____

_____

_____

When I feel good, my life will be different because _____

_____

_____

When I feel good, I will see _____

_____

_____

When I feel good, I will hear _____

_____

_____

What needs to change for you to feel good?

5 of my best personality traits are:

5 skills/abilities I have are:

5 achievements I have attained are:

_____

_____

_____

_____

_____

V. Example letter to younger self

Dear Dan Junior

You are an amazing young boy, who is going through some tough times right now but it won't be forever. These people are wrong to treat you in this way. You deserve better.

Always believe in yourself. You are a good boy. You may do the occasional thing that you shouldn't but that is because you are suffering. Don't be hard on yourself.

Keep believing in yourself. Never listen to anyone who is negative towards you. You can achieve a huge amount. You are smarter than you realise and so capable

You will grow up to be a great man, who will find a good partner in your life. You will have a great career.

I am proud of you, considering everything you have been through, you've come out of it really well. I am your future and you were the amazing lad who gave me this opportunity to live a good life.

I care about you. I love you.

You are amazing.

Dan Senior

VI. Help for suicidal thoughts

When someone feels suicidal, the decision to talk about their feelings is a big step. If you are their chosen confidante, they are likely to feel that you will be understanding and less judgmental than others. Here are some tips on how to have that all-important conversation.

Tips for the chosen confidante:

- If they wish to talk please have patience. Give them time as you sit and listen.

- Ensure you turn off any phone notifications and put your phone on mute. You want to give them your full attention.

- You do not need to have all the solutions. Taking time to listen with empathy is more important right now.

- Do not transfer their feelings onto you and make the conversation about you. E.g. "I felt really down when...."

- They might find it difficult to tell you about their thoughts and feelings but allow them time to talk. Do not feel you need to fill any gaps of silence. They may want to sit in silence with you.

- If, after a while, they feel they cannot talk then try and get them to go for a walk with you or do a normal everyday task with you such as go to the shops or do some DIY. After a while they may open up.

- Ask open questions. Closed ended questions are those which can be answered by a simple 'yes' or 'no'.

Open-ended questions require a more detailed answer. Examples are "what first triggered these feelings?" or "what happened next?"

- Do not make assumptions about their thoughts and feelings. Let them tell you how they have been feeling and what they have been thinking.

- Do your best to ensure they feel heard and their thoughts and feelings are valid, free of judgement even if you do not fully understand.

- Do not try and take this on all by yourself. Talk with them about gaining some professional help. If they agree to this, they may ask you to attend the first session with them and may appreciate you making an initial enquiry. Taking this type of weight of their shoulders is invaluable.

- Use any from the list of contacts provided here or gain insight into who they feel most comfortable talking to. There may be a local therapist who has a good reputation for this type of issue. However, bear in mind many people will not make public that they see a therapist. Some people do not openly share this information. Therefore, you may need to ask a few people for guidance.

VII. Contact details for suicidal support

If you are experiencing suicidal thoughts please contact someone. Here are some contact details (these may be subject to change):

United Kingdom

Go to the Accident & Emergency department at your local hospital

Call 999 and ask for an ambulance if you cannot travel to hospital

Samaritans - freephone 116 123, open 24 hours a day
Visit: https://www.samaritans.org
Email jo@samaritans.org

Campaign Against Living Miserably (CALM) – for men
Call 0800 58 58 58 – 5pm to midnight every day
https://www.thecalmzone.net/help/webchat

Contact your GP for an emergency appointment
NHS 111 (England/Scotland)
NHS Direct 0845 46 47 (Wales)
https://www.england.nhs.uk/contact-us/

Guernsey & Jersey

Samaritans
Freephone: 116 123
Local call charges: Guernsey: (01481) 711030 /
Jersey 0330 094 5717
Email jo@samaritans.org (24-hour response time)

United States

Suicide Prevention Lifeline:
https://suicidepreventionlifeline.org/
SUICIDE: 1-800-784-2433
TALK: 1-800-273-8255
TTY: 800-799-4TTY (4889)
http://suicidehotlines.com/national.html

Boys Town Suicide and Crisis Line (for teens/parents/families)
http://www.boystown.org/national-hotline
1-800-448-3000
Text, Chat Email: http://www.yourlifeyourvoice.org/Pages/ways-to-get-help.aspx

Lifeline Crisis Chat
http://www.crisischat.org
1:1 Online Chat: http://www.crisischat.org/chat
(12:00 pm - 12:00 am EST)

Crisis Text Line
https://www.crisistextline.org/text-us/
Text HOME to 741741 to reach a Crisis Counsellor

VIII. Frequently asked questions

Please remember that I am answering these questions based on my knowledge of the association between mind and body and as a therapist through my experience with clients. These are not based on medical knowledge.

Q. I have no idea where to start if I go to therapy.

A. Do not worry. The therapist will ask some questions to gain some insight into what is happening and progress can be made from there. They may ask you to complete a form before attending your session. Complete the information you feel able to.

You can also use the communication form contained within the Appendix of this book. You could start by considering what is in the way of you enjoying life? The answer might be quite simply a thought or a feeling. Then you have your starting point.

Q. Are some people more pre-disposed to mental health issues?

A. There is not a straightforward response to this question, but in theory, the answer is "yes". We may have a genetic pre-disposition to certain mental health issues. However, just as with any other health issue, we can turn those genes/that DNA on or off. How we live our lives and deal with trauma and stress will have a powerful influence on our ability to never suffer with these illnesses or to manage them in a way that they rarely flare up and live a very good life.

My message to you is whether or not you are aware of family

history, you can take control back of many mental health issues given the right environment and support.

Q. I've heard advice to use a paper bag if you have a panic attack. Is this good advice?

A. More recent advice suggests not to do this and instead ask the person to breathe in and out slowly. Breathe in through their nose and out through their mouth. Someone who suffers with panic attacks may become dependent upon the paper bag. This can cause panic if they do not have a bag readily available. Hence it is best not to become reliant on them.

If someone has other underlying medical conditions, such as asthma or emphysema, using a paper bag may be dangerous for them.

Q. I am not comfortable talking about my problems. What therapies would help me?

A. Most of the therapies I use can be adapted to be content free. In particular Emotional Freedom Technique, Mindfulness Based Inner RePatterning and Matrix Reimprinting can all be adapted. Although not strictly a therapy, Colour Mirrors can also be used in a such a way so that you can keep information solely to yourself. If this is important to you, please check first with the therapist that they are able to work in this way.

In my experience, I have found, once people are comfortable with me, they feel safe to open up and will discuss issues or situations with me they may never have spoken to anyone else about. This does largely come down to your relationship with your therapist of course.

Contact and links

Ann Bowditch
Hypnotherapy & Holistic Health
www.hypnotherapy.gg

YouTube Channel
Ann Bowditch Author

Author Website
Information and supporting documents can be found here.
www.abauthor.com

Wendy Fry
www.wendyfry.com

EFT International
(previously AAMET)
www.EFTInternational.org

General Hypnotherapy Register
www.general-hypnotherapy-register.com

Matrix Reimprinting
www.matrixreimprinting.com

Guild of Energists
www.goe.ac

Rhythmic Movement Training International
www.rhythmicmovement.org

British Association of Urological Surgeons
https://www.baus.org.uk

Other books by Ann Bowditch:

Available from Ann directly or via Amazon:

The Energy of Anxiety
The Power of Confidence

Future books:

Ann will have more books to share in the field of mind, body and emotions. Follow her through her website or via other social media platforms to keep up to date.

Dedication

This book is dedicated to every man struggling with his mental health. You are more capable and powerful than you realise. Use this book to give you the stimulus and motivation to make changes. Take that first step today.

Acknowledgements

Thank you to Jane Bowditch, Dave Edmonds, Jan Marquis, Jo May, Siegi Moherndl, Richard Vahey, Georgie Le Cras, Tara Brehaut and Sam Yabsley for your invaluable feedback. You have been brilliant.

Thank you to Wendy Fry for always being there to offer some advice, encouragement and support.

Printed in Great Britain
by Amazon